THE CASTOR OIL ELIXIR

Rediscover the Healing Power of Castor Oil for a Healthier, Happier You

JENNA JONES

Copyright © 2024 - All rights reserved

No part of this publication may be reproduced, distributed, or transmitted in any form or by any means, including photocopying, recording, or other electronic or mechanical methods, without the prior written permission of the author, except in the case of brief quotations used in reviews or other non-commercial uses permitted by copyright law.

Disclaimer

The information provided in this book is intended for general knowledge and informational purposes only. It is not a substitute for professional medical advice, diagnosis, or treatment. Always seek the advice of a qualified healthcare provider with any questions you may have regarding medical conditions or treatments.

About the Author

Jenna Jones is a dedicated mother and a compassionate nurse with a deep passion for holistic health and natural remedies. With years of experience in healthcare, Jenna has witnessed the powerful effects of both modern medicine and traditional healing methods. Her interest in castor oil grew from a desire to explore safe, natural solutions for her family's well-being.

Drawing on her medical background and personal experiences, Jenna is committed to sharing her knowledge with others who seek to enhance their health through nature's gifts. She believes that the wisdom of ancient remedies, like castor oil, still holds immense value in today's world, especially for those conscious of their health and wellness.

When she's not caring for patients or spending time with her family, Jenna enjoys researching natural therapies, experimenting with DIY wellness recipes, and encouraging others to embrace a balanced, mindful lifestyle.

TABLE OF CONTENTS

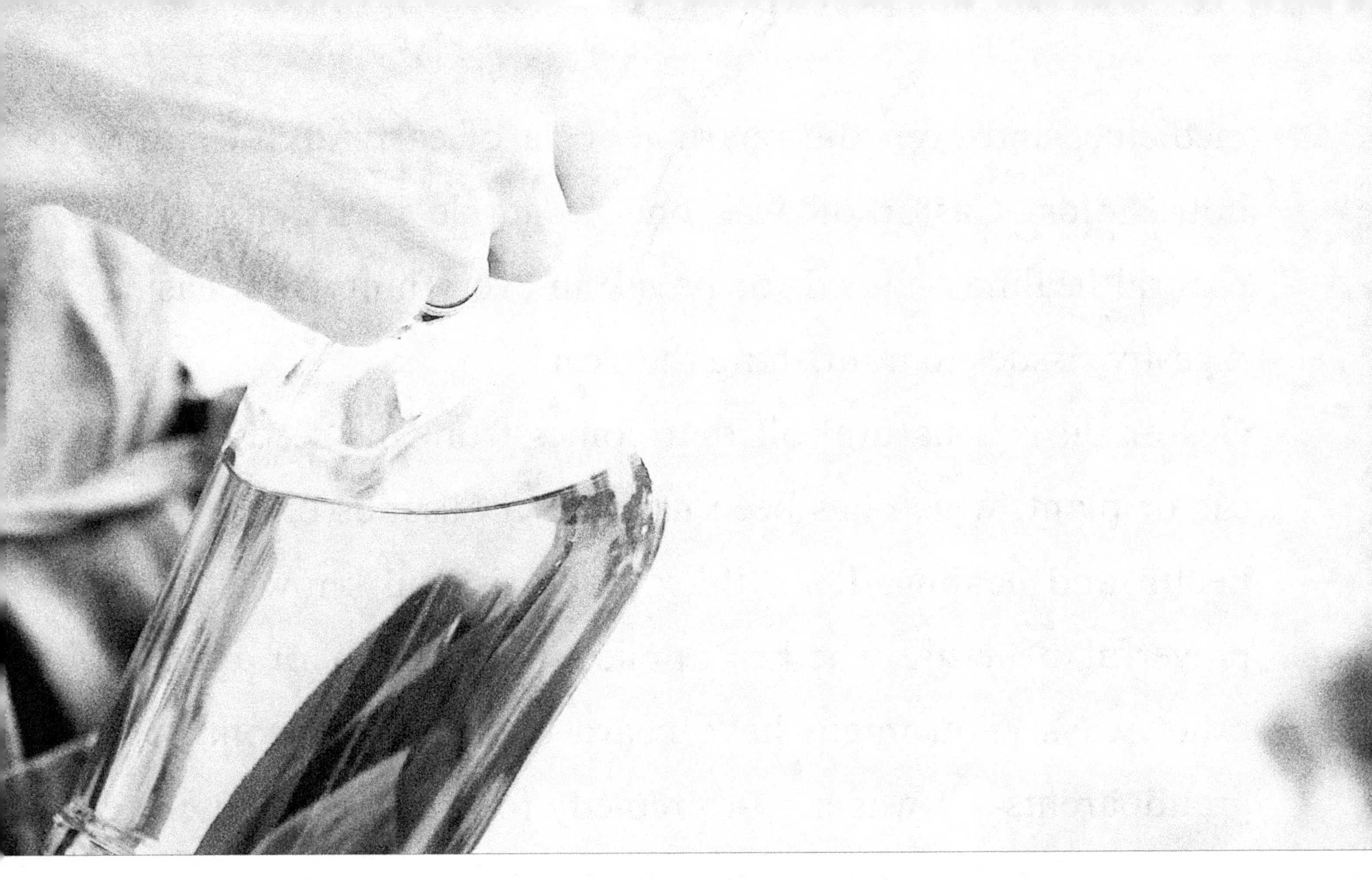

Chapter 1: The Rediscovery of Castor Oil: A Timeless Remedy for Modern Health

What Is Castor Oil?

In the realm of natural remedies, few substances have as rich and varied a history as castor oil. Extracted from the seeds of the castor plant (*Ricinus communis*), this thick, pale-yellow oil has been revered for its powerful health and wellness properties for thousands of years. It has found its place in the annals of ancient Egyptian beauty rituals, Ayurvedic medicine, and even the pharmacopeia of early 20th-century households. Castor oil was once a staple in the world of natural healing—famed for its use in everything from easing digestive issues to nourishing the skin.

Castor oil is a natural oil that comes from the seeds of the castor plant, which has been used for thousands of years for health and healing. It's a thick, yellowish oil known for its powerful benefits, whether applied to the skin or used in other ways. You might have heard of castor oil from your grandparents—it was a go-to remedy for a lot of things, like helping with digestion or healing dry skin. But over time, it has fallen out of everyday use, even though it still has a lot to offer. However, the modern wellness movement is beginning to recognize the value of traditional remedies, and castor oil is once again gaining traction as a versatile, holistic solution for a variety of health concerns.

Why Castor Oil Deserves Your Attention

This book aims to revive the forgotten knowledge of castor oil and highlight why it should be a staple in every health-conscious individual's wellness routine. Whether you're dealing with joint pain, looking to improve the health of your skin and hair, or seeking natural remedies for digestive and menstrual issues, castor oil offers gentle yet powerful solutions that work in harmony with your body.

From scientific research to anecdotal evidence passed down through generations, the benefits of castor oil are both measurable and profoundly personal. Its rich composition of ricinoleic acid, along with other essential fatty acids, gives it unparalleled healing, anti-inflammatory, and moisturizing properties. Moreover, its applications extend beyond personal care—it can be used as an eco-friendly product in the household, for art, and even for sustainable solutions in the environment.

The Purpose of This Book

"The Castor Oil Elixir - Rediscover the Healing Power of Castor Oil for a Healthier, Happier You" is designed to be your comprehensive guide to everything castor oil can do for your health and well-being. This book will take you on a journey through its history, explore its unique properties, and teach you how to incorporate it into your daily routine. You'll find detailed explanations backed by both scientific research and real-life testimonials, as well as practical recipes for using castor oil in skin care, hair care, joint pain relief, and more.

In the chapters that follow, you'll discover simple, effective ways to harness the power of castor oil in your life. We'll delve into topics ranging from how it can detoxify your liver and digestive system to how it can rejuvenate your skin and boost your immune system. And for those looking to make a deep transformation, you'll even find a **30-day detox plan** designed to cleanse and restore balance in your body.

Whether you're new to natural remedies or a seasoned wellness enthusiast, this book is here to guide you in unlocking the full potential of castor oil.

A Historical Journey of Castor Oil

Castor oil's story stretches back thousands of years, across continents and cultures. From the ancient civilizations of Egypt to the traditional healing systems of India, castor oil has been a trusted remedy for various health conditions. Despite its widespread use in the past, this powerful oil fell out of favor in the modern age, replaced by synthetic alternatives and quick fixes. However, as people increasingly return to natural remedies, castor oil is being rediscovered for the healing elixir it has always been.

Ancient Civilizations and Their Use of Castor Oil

Castor oil's earliest known uses date back to ancient Egypt, around 4000 BC. Egyptians valued castor oil for its many benefits, from cosmetic purposes to medicinal applications. It was used as a potent moisturizer in their beauty routines, helping to keep skin soft and hydrated in the harsh desert environment. Castor oil was also used in lamps for lighting and in rituals, where it played a role in purification and embalming. Egyptians were not the only ancient people to embrace the power of castor oil.

In traditional Chinese and Indian medicine, castor oil was widely used for its healing properties. In India, castor oil became a staple in **Ayurveda**, one of the world's oldest holistic healing systems. Ayurvedic practitioners used castor oil to treat digestive issues, boost immunity, and relieve joint pain. Even today, it is used in Ayurvedic practices for its cleansing and detoxifying effects.

Castor Oil in Early Medicine

During the 18th and 19th centuries, castor oil became a household name, particularly in Europe and North America. It was commonly used as a remedy for digestive issues, especially as a natural laxative. Children were often given a spoonful of castor oil to relieve constipation or stomach aches. While the taste was far from pleasant, the results were effective, earning it a place in many family medicine cabinets.

Doctors and pharmacists of the time also recognized castor oil's benefits for skin and wound care. It was applied to cuts and scrapes to speed up healing and reduce infections. Midwives used castor oil to induce labor, and many mothers relied on it as a treatment for colic in babies. By the early 20th century, castor oil had become an essential part of Western medicine, valued for its wide range of uses.

Decline in Modern Times and Its Rediscovery

Despite its long history of success, castor oil saw a decline in popularity in the mid-20th century. The rise of modern pharmaceuticals and synthetic products pushed natural remedies like castor oil to the sidelines. With advancements in medicine, people began to favor quick, over-the-counter solutions, which were often more convenient but sometimes came with side effects.

As castor oil became less common, its rich history and natural benefits were largely forgotten by mainstream society. However, in recent years, the shift towards holistic wellness, sustainability, and chemical-free living has brought castor oil back into the spotlight. People are now rediscovering its incredible versatility and potential, from its ability to heal skin issues and promote hair growth to providing natural relief for joint pain and menstrual discomfort.

In an era where many are seeking healthier, more natural alternatives, castor oil is being revived as a simple, effective solution that works in harmony with the body. No longer just a relic of the past, castor oil is proving to be a valuable tool for modern wellness.

Chapter2: Scientific and Anecdotal Evidence for Castor Oil

Castor oil's wide range of applications has earned it a respected place in traditional healing systems and modern alternative medicine alike. While castor oil has been a staple in natural remedies for centuries, it's only in recent years that science has begun to explore its unique properties more thoroughly. This chapter will take you through the science behind castor oil's effectiveness, backed by both modern research and centuries of anecdotal evidence, offering a complete picture of why this oil is so powerful.

Chemical Composition: The Power of Ricinoleic Acid

The primary active ingredient in castor oil is ricinoleic acid, a rare fatty acid that makes up around 90% of the oil. This compound is largely responsible for castor oil's many health benefits. Unlike other oils, which contain various types of fatty acids, castor oil is unique in its high concentration of ricinoleic acid. Here's how this compound works:

- **Anti-inflammatory properties:** Ricinoleic acid has been shown to reduce inflammation by inhibiting specific enzymes that promote swelling and pain. This makes castor oil particularly effective for joint pain, muscle soreness, and skin inflammation.
- **Antimicrobial action:** Ricinoleic acid has natural antimicrobial properties, meaning it can help fight off bacteria, fungi, and viruses. This explains why castor oil is often used for treating minor wounds, infections, and even acne.
- **Moisturizing effects:** As a humectant, ricinoleic acid draws moisture from the environment into the skin. This makes castor oil a potent natural moisturizer, deeply hydrating the skin while forming a protective barrier to prevent further moisture loss.

Other components found in smaller quantities in castor oil include:

- **Oleic acid**, which enhances skin permeability, allowing deeper absorption of nutrients.

- **Linoleic acid**, known for its anti-inflammatory and skin barrier-repairing properties.
- **Vitamin E**, which acts as an antioxidant, protecting the skin from damage and promoting healing.

How Castor Oil Works: Mechanisms of Action

Topical Applications

Castor oil's ability to penetrate deeply into tissues is one of the reasons it works so effectively when applied to the skin or used in castor oil packs. The oil's high concentration of fatty acids allows it to act as an emollient, softening and nourishing the skin. More than just a surface treatment, castor oil works on deeper layers of the skin, promoting cell regeneration and reducing inflammation.

Internal Use

Castor oil's internal effects are just as impressive, though it must be used with caution. When taken internally, castor oil primarily works as a stimulant laxative. The ricinoleic acid binds to receptors in the intestines, stimulating contractions and pushing waste through the digestive system. This makes it a potent, though occasionally harsh, remedy for constipation. Studies show that castor oil, when consumed in small amounts, can be effective in treating occasional constipation. It works by increasing peristalsis, the muscle contractions that move food through the intestines, leading to bowel movements. Due to its potency, castor oil is generally used internally only under the guidance of a healthcare professional, especially for detoxifying or treating digestive issues.

Modern Research on Castor Oil

Scientific interest in castor oil has grown in recent years, with researchers focusing on its various properties, from wound healing to anti-inflammatory effects. Several key studies offer insight into the oil's therapeutic potential:

- Wound healing properties: A study published in the journal Phytotherapy Research found that castor oil significantly accelerated wound healing. Its antimicrobial and anti-inflammatory effects help in cleaning wounds, reducing infection risk, and promoting faster recovery.
- Anti-inflammatory effects: Research from the Journal of

- Ethnopharmacology suggests that ricinoleic acid has a similar effect to some nonsteroidal anti-inflammatory drugs (NSAIDs), without the harsh side effects. It inhibits the production of pro-inflammatory substances, making it a valuable remedy for chronic inflammation conditions like arthritis.
- Digestive health: Studies on castor oil's use as a laxative have confirmed its effectiveness in promoting bowel movements in people with constipation. However, its potent effect means it should be used sparingly to avoid potential discomfort or dehydration.

While more studies are needed to explore other potential benefits of castor oil, early research supports much of what has been known anecdotally for centuries.

Testimonials and Anecdotal Evidence

For every study conducted on castor oil, there are countless personal stories and experiences passed down through generations. Many of these anecdotes, though not formally researched, paint a compelling picture of castor oil's versatility and effectiveness. Its versatility and effectiveness ranges from skin treatment, hair treatment, acne relief, joint pain and inflammation, chronic arthritis relief, muscle recovery and constipation relief.

The scientific and anecdotal evidence surrounding castor oil paints a clear picture: this ancient remedy is still highly relevant today. Whether backed by research studies or passed down through generations of families, the healing powers of castor oil are difficult to ignore. Ricinoleic acid, castor oil's key component, is the driving force behind its anti-inflammatory, antimicrobial, and moisturizing effects, making it a versatile solution for various health and beauty concerns.

As more people turn away from synthetic treatments in favor of natural, holistic remedies, castor oil is experiencing a well-deserved revival. Its centuries-long track record as a go-to natural remedy is a testament to its enduring power. In the next chapters, we'll explore practical ways to incorporate castor oil into your daily routine, using it for everything from skincare and hair care to joint pain relief and digestive health.

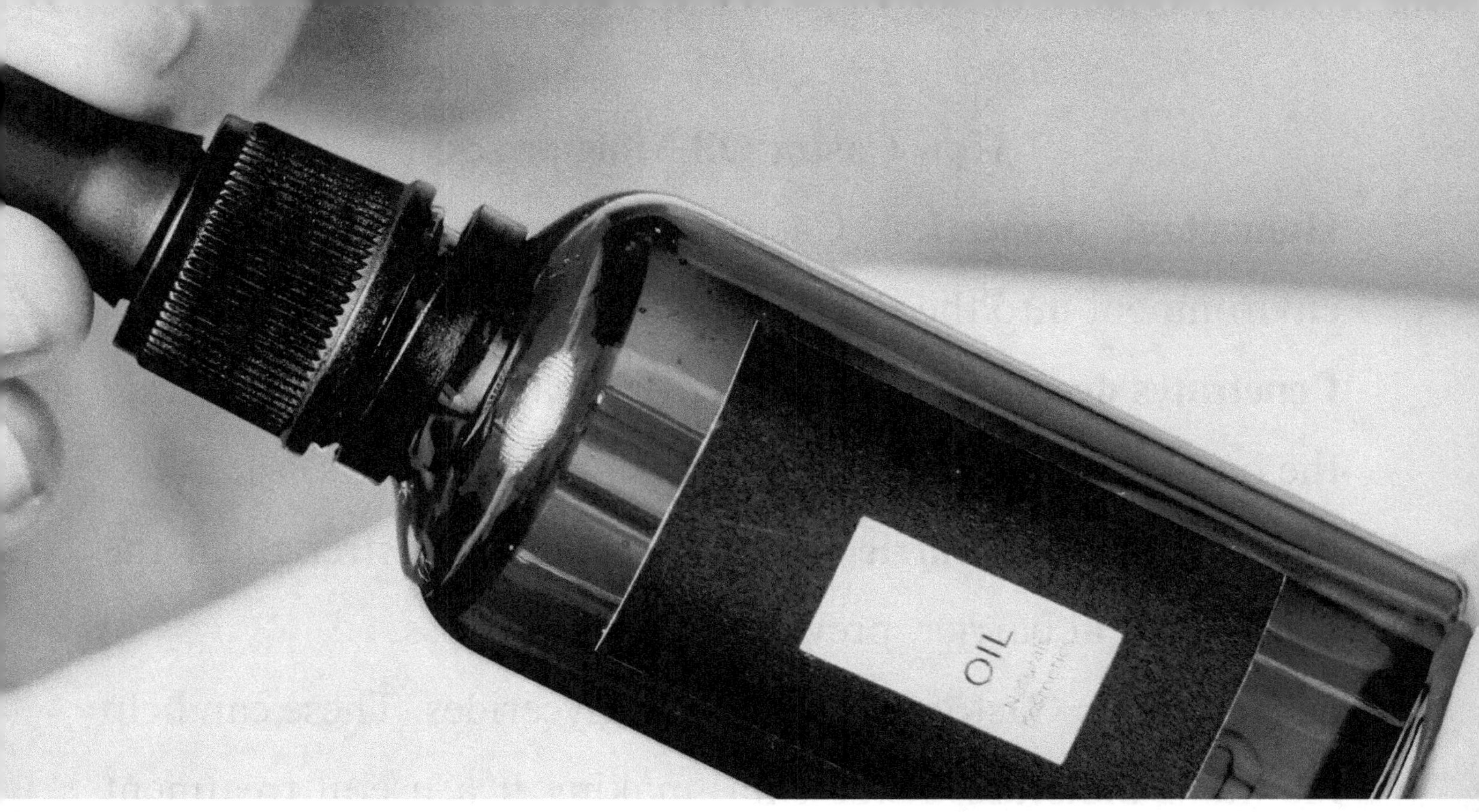

Chapter 3: Comprehensive Skin Care with Castor Oil: From Hydration to Healing

Moisturizing and Nourishing Skin

One of the most common uses of castor oil in skin care is its ability to deeply moisturize. Its thick consistency and humectant properties allow it to draw moisture into the skin and lock it in, making it perfect for individuals with dry or sensitive skin. Castor oil is rich in antioxidants, proteins, vitamin E, and unsaturated fatty acids. It also absorbs easily and repels water, which makes it very efficient at locking moisture in the skin.

How Castor Oil Moisturizes:

Humectant properties: Castor oil draws water from the environment into the skin, providing lasting hydration.

Penetrates deeply: Unlike lighter oils, castor oil can penetrate the outer layer of the skin to nourish deeper tissues.

Protects the skin barrier: Its fatty acids help strengthen the skin's natural barrier, preventing moisture loss.

Moisturizing: Castor oil contains triglycerides. These can help maintain moisture in the skin, making it a useful treatment for dry skin.

Hydration: Castor oil may have humectant properties, which means that it can draw moisture from the air into the skin, keeping the skin hydrated.

Cleansing: The triglycerides found in castor oil are also helpful in removing dirt from the skin.

How to Use Castor Oil for Skin:

Easy DIY Recipe

Castor oil is thick, so you should mix it with a carrier oil before putting it on your face. The recommended ratio is 1:1 – the quantity of castor oil should be the same as the oil with which it is mixed. It can take time for the skin to fully absorb castor oil, but diluting the oil can promote absorption into the skin.

Common carrier oils include:

- coconut oil

- almond oil

- olive oil

You could also add it to shea butter for an extra moisturizing effect. Apply this mixture after cleaning your skin, before bed. You can leave the oil on overnight or wipe it off with a warm cloth after 1 to 5 minutes.

Castor Oil Facial Cleanser and Makeup Remover

Supplies:

- 1 tablespoon Caster oil

- 1 tablespoon Grapeseed or Sweet Almond Oil

- Washcloth

- Combine one tablespoon of castor oil and one tablespoon of sweet almond or grapeseed oil to make a caster oil face cleanser.

- Apply the oil mixture to your face with your fingertips, massaging it into your skin as much as necessary to remove makeup. Give it away liberally, but avoid letting it run.

- Next, use a damp washcloth or organic cotton makeup remover pad to gently wipe your skin. Continue doing this until the washcloth or pad is completely clean and all makeup has been removed.

- Your skin should be completely free of makeup and debris after an oil washing. After that, you can choose to wash your face or go straight to the toning and moisturizing steps.

Castor Oil Nighttime Facial Serum

- 1 tablespoon argan oil
- 1 tablespoon castor oil
- 1 teaspoon rosehip seed oil
- Geranium essential oil

- To create a simple and highly moisturizing facial serum, mix argan oil, castor oil, and rosehip seed oil in a small container and shake well.
- Add a couple of drops of geranium essential oil and mix again for a light, fresh scent.
- Massage serum into facial skin after cleansing and toning before bed.
- Since this is a heavier serum, it's best for nighttime use as it may be too heavy during the day or under makeup.

Sugar Body Scrub With Castor Oil

Supplies:

- 1 cup of plain white granulated sugar or brown sugar
- 1/4 cup of castor oil
- lavender oil

How to:

- Pour one cup of plain white granulated sugar (or brown sugar, if you have it in the pantry; just avoid powdered sugar) into a pint-sized mason jar or other suitable receptacle.
- Next, gradually incorporate 1/4 cup of castor oil into the sugar while stirring. This should be sufficient to cover the white sugar in the cup, but you can always add more oil if you'd like it to be more liquid. Use less oil (or add a little more sugar) if you'd like it a little "dryer".
- Once the desired consistency is achieved, incorporate your preferred essential oils into the mixture. Lavender or ylang-ylang will be more calming, while orange or

lemon are more uplifting.

- Keep your sugar mix covered; if water seeps into the jar while you're showering, it will simply dissolve the sugar, leaving you with a sticky, sugary liquid mess.

Simple Relaxing Massage Oil

- 3 tablespoons castor oil
- Lavender essential oil
- Bergamot essential oil
- Chamomile essential oil

- You can make a calming massage oil for tight shoulders and a sore neck by simply combining castor oil with 5-6 drops of lavender essential oil, 3-4 drops of bergamot essential oil, and 3-4 drops of chamomile essential oil. Mix together in a bottle and shake well.
- To use, rub a few drops of the aromatic oil between your hands and apply to your shoulders and neck to ease tension before going to sleep.

Treating Skin Conditions

Castor oil's anti-inflammatory and antimicrobial properties make it a powerful remedy for various skin conditions, such as acne, eczema, and psoriasis. Its soothing effects can help calm irritated skin and promote faster healing.

Castor Oil For Treating Acne:

Impurities building up in pores leads to the frequent skin ailment known as acne, which is caused by irritated and inflamed skin. Salicylic acid and benzoyl peroxide, two ingredients in many acne treatments available today, have a tendency to dry up the skin.

Simple Relaxing Massage Oil

Supplies:

- A bowl of boiling water
- A towel.
- Washcloth
- Caster oil

- Take a towel and place a bowl of hot water on a level surface. Lean over the bowl of water while holding the cloth over your head. By doing this, you allow the castor oil to deeply infiltrate your skin by opening your pores. Face-down over the bowl for a few minutes.
- Wet a washcloth with warm water, then dab a tiny bit of castor oil onto it the size of a cent. Use the washcloth to gently massage the afflicted area.
- When rubbing castor oil on the affected area, work in little circles.
- Keep the castor oil applied on your skin, overnight. Using a moist towel, wipe away the castor oil as soon as you wake up. Splash your face many times with cold water. Warm water causes your pores to open up, while cold water causes them to contract.
- After patting your skin dry, remove any leftover castor oil with a facial cleanser.
- Repeat these instructions every day for ten to fourteen days to get the best effects. By doing this a few times a week, you can utilize castor oil to avoid acne.

Castor Oil for Oily Skin Recipe

Oily Skin

Oily skin can be a problem for a couple of reasons. The first problem is that oily skin can give your face a shiny appearance, which others may view as unattractive. Additionally, your face will be oily to the touch. The second problem is that the oil on your face can clog your pores. When your pores are clogged, you start forming acne, which gives your skin an unattractive appearance at best and causes permanent scarring at worst.

Supplies:

- Castor Oil (3 Tbsp)
- Sunflower or Extra Virgin Olive Oil (7 Tbsp)

How to:

- Mix castor oil with sunflower or extra virgin olive oil (7 Tbsp)
- Massage the oil blend onto your dry skin for 1-2 minutes.
- Place a warm washcloth over your face to steam the skin and open pores, allowing the oil to penetrate deeply.
- Gently wipe away the oil with the cloth.
- Rinse with cool water and pat your face dry.

Castor Oil for Combination Skin Recipe

Supplies:

- Castor Oil (2 Tbsp)
- Sunflower or Extra Virgin Olive Oil (8 Tbsp)

Combination Skin

When you have combination skin, it means your face is dry in some areas and oily in other areas.

Many people have combination skin. You may have heard of the T-zone (so named because the area looks like a 'T'), which is the central part of the face consisting of the eyes, nose, and mouth. The T-zone is where the skin tends to be oily; the cheeks and area under the eyes might be dry or even flaky.

The recipe to treat combination skin resembles the recipe for oily skin, though you're using less castor oil and more sunflower (or extra virgin olive) oil.

Castor Oil For Dry Skin Recipe

Supplies:

- Castor Oil (1 Tbsp)
- Sunflower or Extra Virgin Olive Oil (9 Tbsp)

Dry Skin

Scaling, itchiness, and cracking characterize dry skin. In general, you're more likely to experience dry skin in the fall and winter months, when the air is dryer. You might also experience it as you get older, as your body produces less oil. More specifically, there are a few lifestyle changes available if you're experiencing dry skin. When you shower, use warm water (rather than hot) as hot water reduces the amount of oil on your skin. After showering, pat the skin dry rather than rub it. Consider showering every other day instead of every day, use soap with moisturizing properties, and apply lotion (also with moisturizing properties) as soon as you get out of the shower.

FOR ECZEMA

In America, eczema is a common inflammatory skin condition that affects 10% of the population. It results in regions of excessively dry, uncomfortable, and itchy skin. Overstretching can disrupt daily living and cause skin infections and blisters. Eczema has no known treatment. On the other hand, flare-ups can be avoided with good skin care, which includes following a regular cleansing and moisturizing routine and avoiding each individual's specific eczema triggers. Prescription and over-the-counter (OTC) drugs can also aid in the management of flare-ups when they happen. Additionally, people with eczema can effectively lessen their symptoms by employing natural therapies, such as oils and gels.

Supplies:

- castor oil
- soft wool or flannel cloth
- olive oil or coconut oil or almond oil

How to:

- Use a small cloth and soak it in the oil mixture.
- Apply the cloth to the area of skin you want to treat.
- Cover the skin using another cloth or plastic sheet, which will help to retain the moisture.

As castor oil is very thick, some people dilute it 1:1 with another oil to allow the skin to absorb it faster.

Potential risks

Castor oil is generally safe when applied to the skin. However, applying undiluted castor oil to the skin may cause mild irritation. Even if it is not a significant irritant, it may cause allergic and severe skin reactions in those with severe eczema and sensitive skin.

Anti-Aging and Wrinkle Prevention

Aging is a natural process that everyone goes through, but there are ways to slow down the visible signs of aging, like wrinkles and fine lines. Castor oil has been praised for its anti-aging properties for generations. Its rich composition of fatty acids and antioxidants makes it a great natural remedy for maintaining youthful, healthy skin.

How Castor Oil Helps Fight Aging

The skin starts to lose its elasticity and hydration as we age, which results in wrinkles, sagging, and dryness. Castor oil can address these issues by nourishing the skin and promoting collagen production, while also protecting it from damage caused by environmental factors like pollution and UV rays.

1. Boosts Collagen Production

Collagen is the protein responsible for keeping skin firm, smooth, and elastic. As we age, collagen production slows down, leading to wrinkles and sagging. Castor oil is rich in ricinoleic acid, which has been shown to stimulate collagen production, helping the skin retain its structure and reduce the appearance of fine lines.

- **Restores elasticity:** Regular use of castor oil helps the skin maintain its elasticity by boosting collagen levels, giving it a firmer, more youthful look.
- **Prevents sagging:** By supporting collagen production, castor oil helps to prevent the sagging that naturally occurs with age, particularly around the eyes and mouth.

2. Deep Hydration for Plumper Skin

One of the key benefits of castor oil is its ability to deeply hydrate the skin. As skin ages, it becomes drier and less able to retain moisture, which can make wrinkles and lines more visible. Castor oil acts as an emollient, softening and hydrating the skin while also sealing in moisture.

- **Locks in moisture:** Castor oil forms a barrier on the skin that prevents water loss, keeping the skin hydrated and plump, which minimizes the appearance of wrinkles.
- **Smoothes fine lines:** By deeply moisturizing the skin, castor oil helps to smooth out fine lines and prevent new ones from forming.

3. Antioxidant Protection Against Free Radical Damage

Free radicals are unstable molecules generated by environmental stressors like sun exposure, pollution, and even stress. These free radicals can damage skin cells, speeding up the aging process and leading to wrinkles, age spots, and dull skin. Castor oil is packed with antioxidants that fight free radical damage and help keep the skin looking youthful.

- **Neutralizes free radicals:** The antioxidants in castor oil, particularly vitamin E, combat oxidative stress caused by free radicals, reducing the formation of new wrinkles.
- **Prevents age spots:** By protecting the skin from sun damage and other environmental factors, castor oil helps

prevent the development of age spots and hyperpigmentation.

How to Use Castor Oil for Anti-Aging

Castor & Aloe Vera Gel Remedy to Reduce the Look of Lines, Wrinkles

Supplies:

- 1 tbsp of aloe vera
- 10 drops of castor oil
- 5 drops of almond oil

Benefits:

According to the Baylor College of Medicine, aloe vera can help with future lines and wrinkles, while almond oil aids with improving complexion, skin tone, and hydration of the skin, and provides a soothing effect.

How to:

- Combine all of the ingredients together until it forms a smooth texture.

- Massage onto your face for 3-5 minutes, using upwards strokes, and then leave on your face for 10 minutes.
- After, remove the mask from your face with warm water or a washcloth.

Oat Flour, Vegetable Glycerin & Castor DIY to Nourish Mature Skin

Supplies:

- 1 tbsp oat flour
- 10 drops of castor oil
- 5 drops of vegetable glycerin
- Water

How to:

- Roughly combine the oat flour, castor oil, and vegetable glycerin, and then gradually add warm water until it forms a smooth paste. If you don't have oat flour, you can grind oats or oatmeal at home using a food processor or blender.
- Using your fingers, apply the mask onto your neck and face and leave on for 12-15 minutes.
- Wash off after

Benefits:

According to a 2017 study, glycerin can effectively relieve dry skin, and another 2017 study indicates that it may also aid in enhancing the skin's barrier function. According to Healthfully, oat flour may aid in moisturizing and softening your skin, which will minimize the look of wrinkles.

Avocado, Apple Juice, Castor Remedy for Firmer Skin

Supplies:

- 1 tbsp of avocado (mashed)
- 8 drops of castor oil
- 10 drops of fresh apple juice

How to:

- Combine all of the ingredients together until it forms a smooth texture. This is a massaging treatment.
- Place a bit of the homemade paste in your hands, and massage onto your face for 3-5 minutes, using upwards strokes, and then leave on your face for 10 minutes.
- After, remove the mask from your face with warm water or a washcloth.

Benefits:

Although everyone enjoys eating avocados and apples, their health advantages extend to our skin in addition to their bellies. Avocado's antioxidants, like vitamin C, can help keep your skin looking youthful by smoothing out wrinkles, WebMD explains, while apple juice works as a natural toner, and hydrates the skin.

Banana, Dark Brown Sugar & Castor Remedy for Glowing & Ageless Skin

Supplies:

- 1 tbsp of banana (mashed)
- 8 drops of castor oil
- 1 tsp of dark brown sugar

How to:

- Combine all of the ingredients together until you can see that the sugar is dissolved.
- This will be a bit more grainy in texture, so pat the mask onto your skin, and massage gently for two minutes around your face and neck, using upward strokes.
- Gently rinse the mask from your face with warm water or a washcloth.

Benefits:

The loss of collagen in the skin is a normal part of aging. Loss of collagen may cause skin to become less sleek and more prone to wrinkles and fine lines. It is believed that a banana's silica can help boost collagen, which can lessen the visibility of wrinkles. In India, bananas are cultivated extensively and utilized for skin care. A natural exfoliator is provided by dark brown sugar.

Healing Scars, Wounds, and Stretch Marks

Healing Scars

Scars can form as a result of injury, surgery, acne, or other skin trauma. While scars are a natural part of the healing process, they can sometimes be unsightly or bothersome. Castor oil can help reduce the appearance of scars by moisturizing the skin, encouraging collagen production, and softening scar tissue.

Why Castor Oil Helps with Scars:

- **Breaks down scar tissue:** Regular application of castor oil helps soften scar tissue, making it more pliable and less noticeable over time.
- **Boosts collagen production:** The increased collagen production stimulated by castor oil improves skin elasticity and helps fill in areas where scars have formed.

Recipe: Castor Oil Scar-Reducing Balm

Supplies:

- 2 tablespoons castor oil
- 1 tablespoon coconut oil
- 5 drops of lavender essential oil
- Mix the oils together and apply to the scar once or twice a day for a soothing, healing balm.

How to:

- Gently massage a small amount of castor oil directly onto the scar twice a day. For deeper penetration, you can cover the area with a warm cloth for 20–30 minutes after application. Consistency is key—results are often visible after several weeks of daily use

Castor Oil for Acne and Scarring

When treating acne with castor oil, you will most probably start to notice results almost immediately. Acne scars can be lightened by using castor oil. Castor oil helps reduce acne and nourish the skin. In addition, it works as an exfoliant, which helps prevent bacteria, oil, dead skin cells, and other toxins from hiding beneath the surface of your skin.

DIY Recipe 1

Supplies:

- 2 tablespoon jamaican black castor oil
- 2 tablespoon grapeseed oil

How to:

- Combine the two oils and apply on the skin. Castor oil is good to lighten acne scars and grapeseed oil can fight acne. This blend will moisturize the skin and is great for cleaning pores on the face.

DIY Recipe 2

Supplies:

- 2 tablespoon jamaican black castor oil
- 2 tablespoon grapeseed oil

- Apply the oil mixture on damaged skin. It helps to remove dead skin layers. It cleanses the skin and helps to keep skin smooth.

DIY Recipe 3

- 3 tablespoon castor seeds oil
- 1 tablespoon multani mitti

- Mix together and apply evenly on your face and let dry. Wash afterwards. This castor oil pack can be used to treat damaged skin cells and regenerate new skin cells in its place. Castor oil improves the healing of acne scars and this oil on acne works wonders!

Safety of Castor Oil and Debunking Concerns

Even though castor oil is beneficial for acne and pimples, you would still need to follow some guidelines and safety precautions before using it. Castor oil can irritate the skin of some people with certain skin conditions.

Therefore, be very careful. Before applying castor oil, make sure that you have thoroughly cleansed your face. Before going to bed at night, you should always rub castor oil on your face. You won't have to worry about acne and pimples appearing on your face.

You should avoid putting unrefined or unfiltered oils directly on your face. Before topical application of castor oil, you should always dilute it with a carrier oil or moisturizer first.

Treating Minor Wounds

Castor oil's antimicrobial and anti-inflammatory properties make it an excellent remedy for minor cuts, scrapes, and burns. It not only helps prevent infection but also speeds up the healing process by keeping the wound moist and protected.

How Castor Oil Aids Wound Healing:

Prevents infection: Castor oil has antimicrobial properties that can help prevent bacteria from infecting the wound.

Keeps the wound moist: A key aspect of wound healing is maintaining moisture. Castor oil acts as a protective barrier, preventing the wound from drying out and forming a scab too early, which can reduce the likelihood of scarring.

Minor Wounds

- 1 tablespoon of cold-pressed castor oil

- 2-3 drops of tea tree essential oil (optional for extra antibacterial properties)

- 1 teaspoon of coconut oil (optional for added moisture and healing)

- Sterile cotton balls or gauze pads

- Adhesive bandage (if needed)

How to:

- Gently clean the wound with mild soap and water to remove dirt, debris, or bacteria. Pat the area dry with a clean towel. In a small bowl, mix 1 tablespoon of castor oil with 2-3 drops of tea tree essential oil (optional) for its antibacterial properties. If you prefer a more moisturizing blend, add 1 teaspoon of coconut oil.

- Using a sterile cotton ball or gauze pad, apply a thin layer of the castor oil mixture directly to the wound. Make sure the entire affected area is covered with the oil.

- If the wound is in an area that might be exposed to dirt or friction, cover it with a sterile adhesive bandage or gauze pad to protect it. If the wound is in a low-risk area, you may leave it uncovered to allow air to promote healing.

Note: Castor oil should only be used on minor wounds. For deeper or more serious injuries, always seek medical attention first.

Reducing Stretch Marks

Stretch marks, or striae, are a common concern for many people, especially during pregnancy, rapid weight gain or loss, and puberty. They occur when the skin stretches rapidly, causing the collagen and elastin fibers to break down. While stretch marks are natural and pose no health risks, many people seek ways to reduce their appearance.

Why Castor Oil is Effective for Stretch Marks:

Deeply moisturizes: Castor oil penetrates deep into the skin, providing intense hydration that helps keep the skin soft and supple. This deep moisture can reduce the visibility of existing stretch marks and help prevent new ones from forming.

Improves elasticity: By boosting collagen production, castor oil helps restore skin elasticity, making it more resilient to further stretching.

Fades marks over time: With regular use, castor oil can help lighten and smooth stretch marks, making them less noticeable.

Castor Oil Stretch Mark Serum

Supplies:

- 2 tablespoons castor oil
- 1 tablespoon almond oil or coconut oil
- 10 drops of vitamin E oil
- Massage this serum into areas with stretch marks daily to help fade them and improve skin elasticity.
- Plastic wrap (for optional heat therapy)
- Warm towel or heating pad (optional)

How to:

- In a small bowl, mix 2 tablespoons of castor oil with 1 tablespoon of coconut oil. Add 3-4 drops of vitamin E oil to boost the skin's healing and moisturizing properties. Stir the oils together until well-blended.

- Massage the oil mixture into the skin over the areas affected by stretch marks (e.g., thighs, abdomen, hips, or arms). Use gentle, circular motions for 5-10 minutes, ensuring the oil is thoroughly absorbed into the skin.
- For deeper penetration and enhanced results, you can use heat therapy. After massaging the oil, wrap the area with plastic wrap to keep the moisture locked in. Place a warm towel or heating pad over the wrapped area for 20-30 minutes. This heat will allow the castor oil to penetrate more deeply into the skin and boost its effectiveness.
- Repeat Regularly:For best results, repeat this treatment daily, preferably after a shower or before bed, when the skin is clean and ready to absorb the oil. Consistency is key—results may take several weeks to become noticeable.

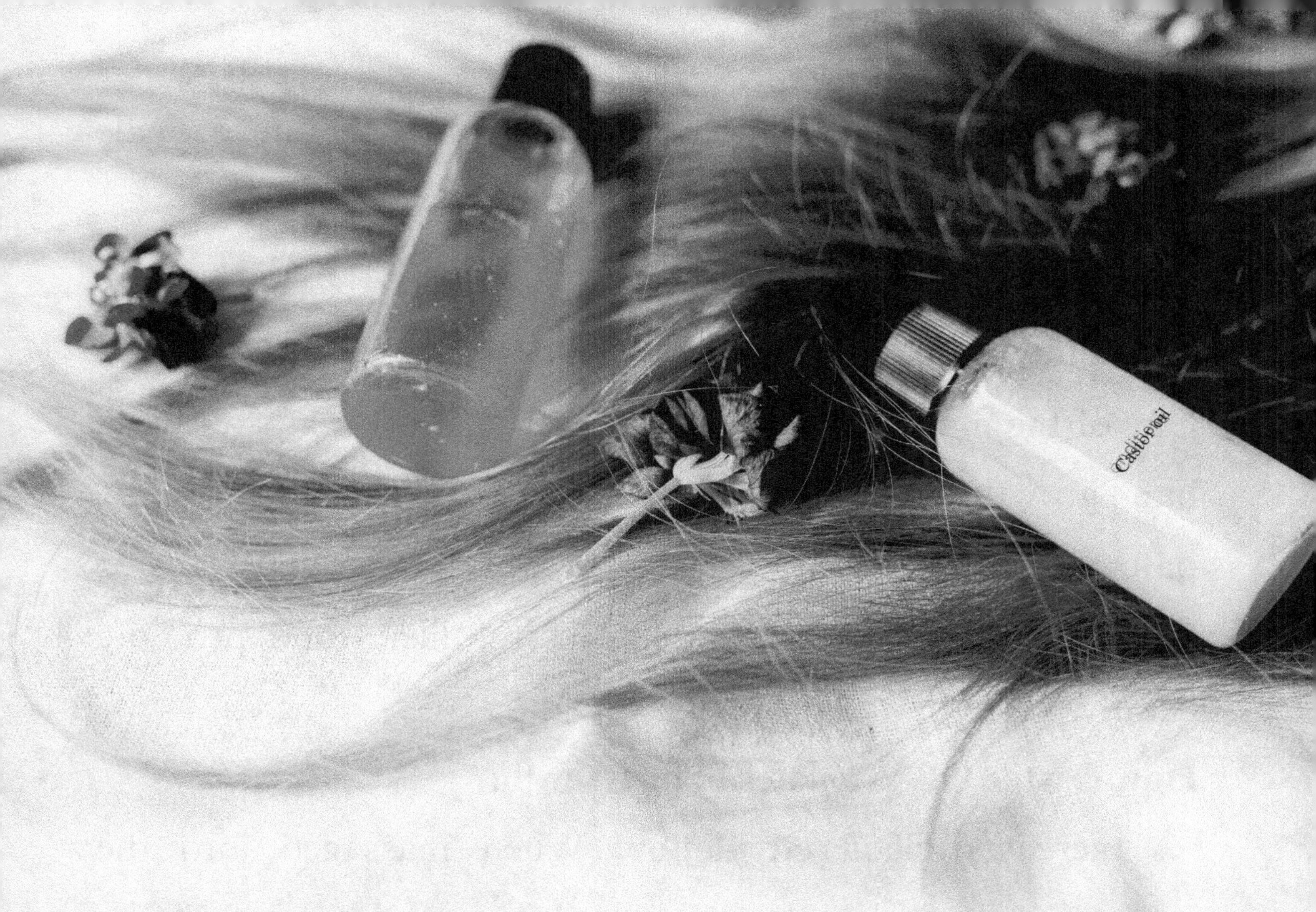

Chapter 4: Castor Oil for Ultimate Hair Care: Growth, Strength, and Scalp Health

When it comes to natural hair care, castor oil is a powerhouse. Its thick, nutrient-rich composition makes it ideal for nourishing the scalp, strengthening hair, and promoting growth. Whether you're looking to improve the condition of your hair, address hair loss, or simply boost shine and softness, castor oil can play a key role in transforming your hair's health. In this chapter, we'll explore the many ways castor oil can benefit your hair and provide practical tips and recipes for using it effectively.

Promoting Hair Growth

One of the most popular uses of castor oil is for encouraging hair growth. Whether you're experiencing hair thinning, patchy spots, or just want to boost overall hair length, castor oil has been shown to stimulate hair follicles and promote healthy growth.

How Castor Oil Promotes Hair Growth:

- **Increases blood circulation:** When massaged into the scalp, castor oil increases blood flow to the hair follicles, ensuring they receive more nutrients and oxygen, which supports hair growth.
- **Strengthens hair roots:** The rich ricinoleic acid in castor oil has nourishing properties that strengthen the roots of the hair, reducing hair breakage and fall.
- **Fights scalp infections:** Castor oil's antifungal and antibacterial properties help protect the scalp from infections that can hinder hair growth, such as dandruff or scalp dermatitis.

Hair Growth Booster Serum

- 2 tablespoons castor oil
- 2 tablespoons coconut oil
- 10 drops rosemary essential oil

- Mix the oils together and massage into your scalp 1–2 times a week. Rosemary oil is known for stimulating hair growth, while coconut oil helps moisturize the scalp.
- Massage it into your scalp using circular motions. Allow it to sit for at least 30 minutes, or leave it on overnight for a more intense treatment. Rinse thoroughly with shampoo.

Castor Oil for Hair Loss

You can apply castor oil for hair loss in a manner similar to how you would for hair growth. If you've suddenly been experiencing more hair loss, you can lean on castor oil's nourishing ingredients to strengthen the strand. Vitamin E and protein are stars here: both known for repairing the tissues of our body and readily available when using castor oil for hair loss!

- 1 tablespoon of caster oil
- 1 tablespoon of peppermint oil or Rosemary oil

- Pair your castor oil with peppermint oil and/or rosemary oil. Why? Peppermint oil is known to increase the depth of follicles. While rosemary oil is scientifically proven to combat the hair-thinning hormone dihydrotestosterone in your follicle.
- Massage it into your scalp using circular motions. Allow it to sit for at least 30 minutes, or leave it on overnight for a more intense treatment. Rinse thoroughly with shampoo.

Castor Oil Hair Serum Recipe

A mix of castor oil and jojoba will make a hair serum to help your hair grow faster, stronger, and smoother.

- 3 tablespoons of caster oil
- 1 tablespoon of jojoba oil or argan oil

- Mix the ingredients and shake to mix.
- Apply to the scalp.
- Then, massage for 5 minutes to make sure the entire scalp is coated and to help increase circulation.

Castor Oil Hair Masks For Maximized Hair Growth (Shiny and Strong)

1. Castor oil, tea tree and aloe vera hair mask

The healing and soothing properties of aloe vera and caster oil hair masks are ideal for rejuvenating your scalp and regulating the healthy sebum, an oily substance that keeps hair from drying and breaking off. Moreover, tea tree oil has antiseptic, antiviral, and antifungal properties that kill harmful microbes, thus promoting hair growth.

Supplies:

- 2 tablespoons castor oil
- ½ cup of aloe vera gel
- 2-3 drops of tea tree oil

- In a bowl, mix castor oil with aloe vera gel. Stir well to convert it into a paste.
- Then, add tea tree oil drops to the past and continue mixing the ingredients for at least 2-3 minutes.
- Now, gently apply this paste to your hair and scalp. Remember to wear a shower cap and let the mask set properly.
- Keep the mask for 30-40 minutes, and then wash it off using a mild shampoo with normal-temperature water. Use the mask at least twice a week.

2. Castor oil, almond oil and fenugreek hair mask

Castor oil helps to lubricate the hair shaft, increase flexibility and decrease the chances of breakage. On the other hand, fenugreek is rich in iron and protein, nutrients essential for hair growth. These ingredients together make for a perfect combination to promote hair growth.

Supplies:

- 3 tablespoons castor oil
- 1 tablespoon fenugreek powder
- 1 tablespoon almond oil

How to:

- Take a bowl and add fenugreek powder and mix it with castor and almond oil. Mix these ingredients till you see a paste-like consistency.
- Apply this paste across the length of your hair, dip a towel in warm water, and wrap it around your hair for 10-15 minutes.
- Keep the mask on for another 30-40 minutes, and then rinse using a mild shampoo. For optimum benefits, apply the mixture twice a week to help your hair grow faster.

3. Castor oil, honey and egg hair mask

The nourishing properties of eggs combined with the strengthening properties of castor oil and honey's cleansing abilities make this hair mask a perfect hair care treatment.

Supplies:

- 2 tablespoons castor oil
- 1 tablespoon honey
- 1 egg

- Whisk the egg in a bowl and combine it with honey and castor oil. Add water if required for consistency and volume.
- Now, mix all the ingredients and then start applying to your hair roots and strands.
- Cover your hair with a shower cap and let it sit for at least an hour before rinsing it with cold water and a mild shampoo. Using this mask at least twice a week will help restore and maintain the hair's health.

Thickening Hair

In addition to promoting growth, castor oil can also help thicken hair. This is especially beneficial for people with thin, fine hair who are looking for more volume and density.

Why Castor Oil Thickens Hair:

Nourishes hair strands: Castor oil's fatty acids coat each strand of hair, giving it a thicker, fuller appearance while also making the hair stronger.

Prevents breakage: By hydrating and nourishing the hair shaft, castor oil reduces breakage and split ends, which helps maintain hair density.

Supplies:

- 1 tablespoon of caster oil
- I tablespoon of olive oil or almond oil

How to:

- Mix equal parts castor oil and olive oil (or a lighter oil like almond oil), and apply it to the length of your hair, focusing on the ends. Leave it on for 30 minutes to an hour before washing it out.
- Use this treatment once a week for visibly thicker, fuller hair over time.

OR

Supplies:

- 1 tablespoon of caster oil
- 1 tablespoon of argan oil
- Rosemary essential oil

How to:

- Combine 1 tablespoon of castor oil with 1 tablespoon of argan oil and a few drops of rosemary essential oil. Argan oil nourishes the hair, while rosemary essential oil is famed for promoting hair growth.
- Apply to the scalp, leave it on for an hour or overnight, then wash out.

Moisturizing Dry and Damaged Hair

Dry, damaged hair can result from heat styling, harsh hair products, or environmental factors like sun and wind. Castor oil's intense moisturizing properties help restore dry hair to its natural softness and shine by sealing in moisture and nourishing the hair shaft from within.

How Castor Oil Repairs Damaged Hair:

- **Deeply hydrates hair:** Castor oil penetrates the hair shaft, locking in moisture to keep hair hydrated and preventing further damage from dryness.
- **Repairs split ends:** By coating and protecting the hair, castor oil helps to smooth split ends and prevent further breakage.

Supplies:

- castor oil
- 1 tablespoon honey
- 1 tablespoon coconut oil, argan oil or jojoba oil

How to:

- Apply a generous amount of castor oil to the ends of your hair, or wherever it feels dry or damaged. Mix castor oil with argan or jojoba oil and leave it on for 1–2 hours, or overnight for very dry hair, before washing it out.

- This treatment can be done once a week for intense repair or every other week for maintenance.

Treating Scalp Conditions (Dandruff)

A healthy scalp is the foundation of healthy hair. Castor oil's antimicrobial and anti-inflammatory properties make it an excellent remedy for a range of scalp conditions, from dandruff to fungal infections. It helps soothe irritation, fight infections, and restore balance to the scalp, which in turn promotes healthier hair growth.

How Castor Oil Treats Common Scalp Problems

Fights dandruff: Castor oil's antifungal properties help eliminate dandruff-causing fungi, while its moisturizing effects prevent the scalp from becoming too dry or flaky.

Soothes scalp irritation: Its anti-inflammatory properties can help calm irritated, itchy, or inflamed skin on the scalp.

Balances oil production: Regular use of castor oil can help balance the scalp's natural oil production, reducing excess oiliness or dryness.

Recipe: Dandruff Treatment Oil

- 2 tablespoons castor oil
- 1 tablespoon olive oil
- 5 drops tea tree essential oil

- Mix and apply to the scalp, leaving it on for 30–60 minutes before rinsing thoroughly. Repeat once a week to control dandruff and soothe the scalp.

Castor Oil, Aloe Vera Gel, And Tea Tree Oil

Castor and tea tree oil help fight against dandruff. Aloe vera gel acts as a soothing agent and reduces scalp itchiness.

- Castor oil, 1 ½ tablespoons
- Aloe vera gel, 3 tablespoons
- Tea tree oil, 2 to 3 drops

- Mix the three oils in a bowl apply the mixture to your scalp Leave it on for about 45 minutes, cover your head with a shower cap.

- Wash with an herbal shampoo, follow this routine thrice a week.

Castor Oil, Almond Oil, And Rosemary Oil

Like castor oil, almond oil also helps prevent dandruff by moisturizing your scalp. Almond oil is rich in vitamin E, which may help moisturize your hair. Rosemary oil may exhibit antifungal activity against dandruff.

Supplies:

- Castor oil, 1 tablespoon
- Almond oil, 1 tablespoon
- Rosemary oil, 2 to 3 drops

How to:

- Mix the castor and almond oils in a glass bowl.
- Heat the mixture in a microwave oven for a few seconds.
- Add rosemary oil to the mixture.
- Apply this mixture to your hair and scalp. Leave it on overnight.
- Follow this routine thrice a week.

Castor Oil And Ginger Juice

Ginger juice may seem like a stinky ingredient to put on your hair, but it can do a world of good to your hair. Anecdotal evidence suggests that ginger juice can clear clogged pores and cleanse away dandruff, dirt, and product buildup

Supplies:

- Castor oil, 2 tablespoons
- Ginger juice, 2 tablespoons

How to:

- Mix the castor oil and ginger juice. Apply this mixture to your scalp, leave it on for 30 minutes. Wash with an herbal shampoo. Follow this routine thrice a week.

Castor Oil And Argan Oil

Using argan oil on your head can help get rid of your dandruff and give you softer hair. The moisturizing properties of argan oil may help treat dandruff, tame down the frizz, and make your hair look shinier. However, more research is needed in this regard.

- Castor oil, 2 tablespoons
- Argan oil, 1 tablespoon

- Mix the oils in a glass bowl. Heat the mixture in a microwave for a few seconds. Apply the mixture to your scalp and hair. Leave it on overnight. Wash with a mild shampoo.
- Follow this routine twice a week.

Castor Oil, Coconut Oil, And Egg

Castor and coconut oils work synergistically well to deeply condition your scalp. Coconut oil has a high affinity for hair proteins and can easily penetrate the hair shaft. Its penetrating powers may get the required nutrients into your hair shaft, preventing a dry scalp, hair loss, and dandruff. Research shows that the application of coconut oil may prevent severe dandruff. The protein from the egg nourishes your hair and makes it soft and shiny.

- Castor oil, 1 tablespoon
- Coconut oil, 1 tablespoon
- Egg, 1

- Whisk the egg and castor and coconut oils in a bowl. Apply this mixture to your scalp and hair. Leave it on for 30 minutes. Wash with cool water and a mild shampoo.
- Follow this routine once a week.

Castor Oil And Olive Oil

Olive oil is a renowned natural hair conditioner. In contrast to conventional store-bought conditioners that may potentially congest and irritate your scalp, olive oil effectively moisturizes a dry scalp and alleviates flakiness.

- 2 tablespoons of castor oil
- 2 tablespoons of olive oil

- Mix both the oils in a bowl. Heat up the blend slightly to make it lukewarm. Apply this warm oil blend to your scalp and gently massage it in with your fingertips in small, circular motions. Leave it on for at least 30 minutes or overnight.
- Shampoo your hair with your regular shampoo and warm water. Do a final rinse with cold water.
- Use this treatment once a week

Enhancing Hair Shine and Smoothness

For those looking to add extra shine and smoothness to their hair, castor oil is a great solution. Its thick, viscous nature helps to coat the hair, adding a protective layer that reflects light and gives hair a glossy, healthy appearance.

How Castor Oil Enhances Shine

- **Coats the hair shaft:** Castor oil forms a protective layer over each strand, smoothing the hair cuticle and creating a glossy finish.
- **Prevents frizz:** By sealing in moisture, castor oil helps tame frizz and flyaways, leaving hair looking smooth and sleek.

Shine-Enhancing Hair Serum

- 1 tablespoon castor oil
- 1 tablespoon argan oil
- 5 drops of lavender essential oil
- Mix and apply a few drops to damp or dry hair to boost shine and smooth frizz.

- Rub a small amount of castor oil between your palms and lightly smooth it over the length of your hair after styling, focusing on the ends. Be careful not to use too much, as it can weigh the hair down.
- For a more intense shine treatment, use castor oil as a pre-wash hair mask. Apply it from root to tip and leave it on for 1-2 hours before shampooing.

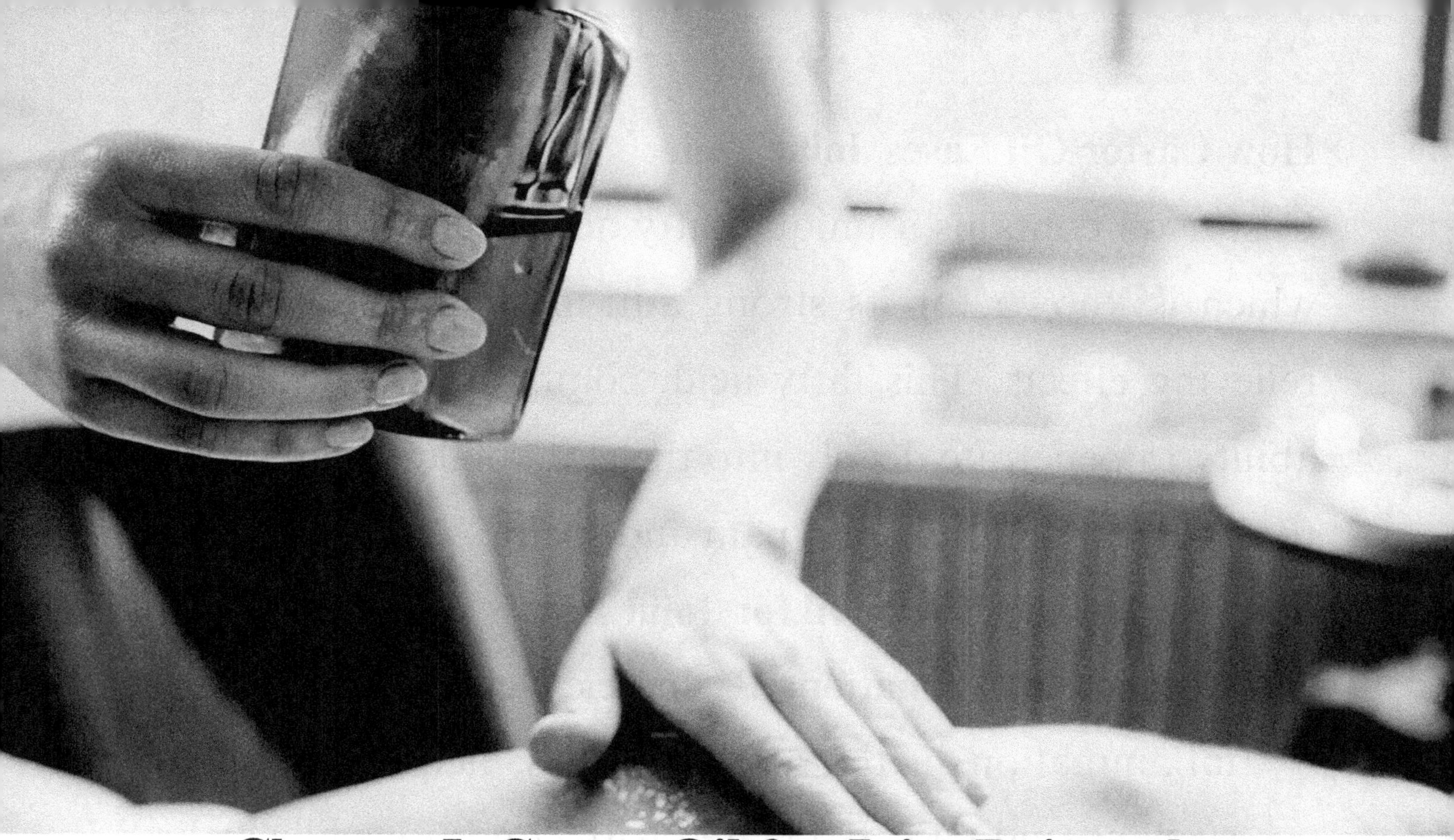

Chapter 5: Castor Oil for Joint Pain and Inflammation: Natural Relief for Arthritis and Muscle Stiffness

Joint pain and inflammation can significantly impact one's quality of life, especially for individuals dealing with chronic conditions like arthritis or muscle stiffness from injuries. While conventional treatments often focus on medications and physical therapy, natural remedies like castor oil have been used for centuries to offer relief. Castor oil's potent anti-inflammatory and analgesic properties make it an effective and accessible option for those seeking natural solutions to reduce pain and promote joint health.

How Castor Oil Eases Joint Pain

Castor oil contains a unique fatty acid called ricinoleic acid, which is known for its strong anti-inflammatory and pain-relieving effects. This fatty acid, combined with castor oil's ability to penetrate deeply into the skin, makes it an excellent topical treatment for joint pain and stiffness.

Key Benefits of Castor Oil for Joint Pain:

- **Reduces inflammation:** Ricinoleic acid works to reduce inflammation in the affected areas, helping to alleviate swelling and pain associated with conditions like arthritis or injury.

- **Improves circulation:** When applied topically, castor oil helps increase blood flow to the joints, which can enhance mobility and reduce stiffness.

- **Relaxes muscles:** The oil's soothing properties can also help relax muscles surrounding the joints, providing relief from tension and improving joint flexibility.

Common Conditions Treated with Castor Oil

Castor oil can be beneficial for various conditions that cause joint pain or inflammation. Here are a few common ailments where castor oil has been used effectively:

Arthritis

Arthritis is a condition marked by inflammation of the joints, causing pain, swelling, and reduced mobility. Castor oil's anti-inflammatory properties make it an excellent remedy for arthritis pain, particularly for conditions like osteoarthritis and rheumatoid arthritis.

Castor Oil Rub For Arthritis Pain Relief

Supplies:

- Castor oil
- Cotton Pads

How to:

- Warm up castor oil, not too hot but just a little warm, and soak cotton pads in castor oil.
- Take a little at a time and thoroughly massage the oil all over the skin on the arthritis-affected area, and place a hot water pack or hot water bottle there. This castor oil massage therapy is good for conditions like general joint stiffness and reducing severe pain and inflammation. Use it at least twice a week for arthritis.

Castor Oil Pack For Arthritis

Supplies:

- Castor Oil
- Hot water pack (bag or pads).
- Cotton pads

Prep Time

- 8 Hours

Processing Time

- 1 hour

How to:

- For chronic arthritis pain and joint pain, you can soak a cotton pad or two in castor oil overnight, squeeze off the excess, and massage with a hot water pack or hot water bottle over the affected area.
- Continue applying this organic remedy every week or once in two weeks at least, depending on the intensity of arthritis pain and inflammation.

Castor oil And Orange Juice For Arthritis

Supplies:

- Castor oil
- One glass of orange juice

How to:

- Take about one to two teaspoons of castor oil and boil it. Once it is warm enough, add this lukewarm castor oil to a glass of orange juice, preferably fresh.

NOTE: This remedy works effectively on people on an alkaline diet. Also, make sure you consult your doctor about any dietary supplements or restrictions for maximum benefits.

Castor Oil In Ginger Tea For Arthritis

Supplies:

- Ginger
- Tea powder
- Castor oil
- Water

Prep Time

- 5 minutes

How to:

- Pour tea into water as you normally would.
- Grate the ginger into boiling water and let it simmer over medium heat for 5-10 minutes.
- Turn off the stove after the water simmers and filter the pulp.
- If you are making it for more than a cup, add 1-2 teaspoons of castor oil for each extra serving.
- This is an excellent remedy to relieve arthritic pain and inflammation. It also helps you sleep better.

NOTE: Castor oil has laxative properties, so people with sensitive bowel syndrome, diarrhea, and other digestive health issues might want to avoid this remedy.

How Often: Depending on the intensity of your joint pain, take this remedy at least two or three times a week for maximum benefits.

Castor Oil And Flannel Pack

Supplies:

- Cotton flannel cloth
- Castor oil (for topical use)
- Plastic/cling wrap
- Towel
- Hot water bottle or hot water pack

Prep Time

- 5 minutes

Processing Time

- 45 minutes
- 1 hour

How to:

- Take about 20 ml of castor oil and warm it over the stove or just microwave it.
- Fold the flannel and soak it in castor oil. Leave it on for about 20 minutes till the flannel completely absorbs the oil.
- Place a piece of cloth or towel over the affected painful joint to keep it elevated and protect the skin from excess heat.
- Wrap the arthritis-affected area with the flannel cloth soaked in castor oil.

- Now, wrap the cotton flannel cloth with plastic or cling wrap for binding it all intact.
- Leave this castor oil pack for at least 30-45 minutes.
- It could be a little messy, so ensure there's no oil spillage around the house, or it's best you sit outdoors or on the balcony while you use this castor oil wrap.

How Often?

Apply this natural remedy at least 2-3 days consecutively.

Give it a break and continue after a week or so.

You could bring it down to 15-20 minutes as you start feeling relieved from stiffness and inflammation.

Muscle Stiffness and Soreness

After intense physical activity or prolonged periods of inactivity, muscles can become stiff and sore. Castor oil helps relax these tense muscles, reducing pain and stiffness.

How to use: Massage castor oil onto the sore or stiff muscles. You can also add a few drops of peppermint or eucalyptus essential oil for additional cooling and soothing effects.

Tendonitis and Bursitis

Both tendonitis (inflammation of a tendon) and bursitis (inflammation of the fluid-filled sacs that cushion the joints) can cause significant discomfort. Castor oil's ability to reduce inflammation can bring relief from the pain and swelling caused by these conditions.

How to use: Apply castor oil directly to the inflamed area and gently massage. Follow up with a warm cloth or heating pad to increase circulation and ease discomfort.

Castor Oil Packs for Joint Pain Relief

A castor oil pack is a piece of wool or a cloth soaked in castor oil that you can apply on the skin. One of the most effective ways to use castor oil for joint pain is through the application of castor oil packs. These packs help deliver the oil's healing properties directly to the affected area, maximizing its benefits. The heat from the pack enhances absorption and promotes circulation, further easing inflammation and stiffness.

Instructions to make a castor oil pack

Supplies:

- castor oil
- unbleached wool or cotton flannel
- medium container or bowl
- tongs
- scissors
- plastic sheeting, such as a small tablecloth or garbage bag

- Cut the wool or cotton flannel into rectangular pieces, about 12 inches by 10 inches. You can also cut them into strips or smaller squares depending on where you'll use them.
- Use at least three to four pieces of cloth to make a pack.
- Pour castor oil into the container. You should be able to completely soak a piece of the wool or cotton flannel in the castor oil.
- Drop one piece of the cloth into the oil until it's completely soaked.
- Use the tongs to pick up the cloth in the container. It should be dripping with castor oil.
- Lay the soaked cloth flat on the plastic sheet.
- Soak the other two or more pieces of cloth in the same way.
- Add the oil-soaked cloths flat on top of the first one.
- Once you've soaked and layered each cloth, you've made a castor oil pack.

Using Castor Oil for Knee Joint Pain Relief

Combining Castor Oil and Turmeric

Turmeric, known for its potent anti-inflammatory properties, can be an effective complement to castor oil in alleviating knee joint pain. A mixture of castor oil and turmeric can be used for massaging the affected area to reduce pain and inflammation.

Here's a simple recipe for a castor oil and turmeric mixture:

- Combine two tablespoons of castor oil with a teaspoon of turmeric powder.
- Mix well until a paste is formed.
- Apply this mixture to the knee joint, gently massaging it into the skin.
- Allow it to sit for 15-20 minutes before washing off with warm water.
- This combination harnesses the anti-inflammatory properties of both castor oil and turmeric, providing a natural and effective remedy for knee joint pain.

Blending Castor Oil with Essential Oils

Essential oils, particularly peppermint oil, can also be combined with castor oil to alleviate knee joint pain. Peppermint oil is known for its analgesic and anti-inflammatory properties, making it a valuable addition to the castor oil.

A blend of castor oil and peppermint oil can be massaged onto the knee joint to help relieve pain.

Here's how to create this blend:
- Combine two tablespoons of castor oil with five drops of peppermint essential oil.
- Stir well until the oils are thoroughly mixed.
- Apply this blend to the knee joint, gently massaging it into the skin in circular motions for a few minutes.
- Leave it on for at least 30 minutes before washing off with warm water.

This mixture capitalizes on the anti-inflammatory benefits of castor oil and the analgesic properties of peppermint oil, providing an effective, natural solution for knee joint pain. Remember to always conduct a patch test when using any new essential oils to avoid potential skin irritations.

Using castor oil for knee joint pain relief can be an effective natural remedy. However, it's important to remember that these methods should be used as a complementary treatment and not replace medical advice or prescribed treatments. Always consult with a healthcare provider before starting any new treatment regimen.

Combining Castor Oil with Other Remedies

While castor oil is powerful on its own, combining it with other natural remedies can amplify its effects on joint pain and inflammation.

1. Castor Oil and Ginger

Ginger is well known for its anti-inflammatory properties, and when combined with castor oil, it can provide even more effective pain relief.

How to use: Grate a small piece of fresh ginger and mix it with a few tablespoons of castor oil. Heat the mixture slightly, then apply it to the affected joint. Massage gently and cover with a warm cloth for enhanced relief.

2. Castor Oil and Epsom Salt Baths

Epsom salt is rich in magnesium, which can help reduce inflammation and ease muscle tension. Combining castor oil with an Epsom salt bath provides soothing relief for sore joints and muscles.

How to use: Add 1–2 cups of Epsom salt to a warm bath along with 2 tablespoons of castor oil. Soak in the bath for 20–30 minutes to relieve joint pain and relax muscles.

Scientific Evidence Supporting Castor Oil for Joint Pain

Several studies have supported the use of castor oil in reducing inflammation and pain, particularly for joint-related issues:

- A number of research papers and clinical trials support the use of castor oil as a knee joint pain reliever. A 2008 study indicated that castor oil pack therapy was effective in treating osteoarthritis pain in the knees. The report was published in Complementary Therapies in Clinical Practice. After just seven days of treatment, the participants reported a considerable improvement in their discomfort.

- In a 2011 clinical trial, the International Quarterly Journal of Research in Ayurveda (AYU) reported that, over the course of a 15-day study period, administering 30 to 40 ml of castor oil with hot water to patients with rheumatoid arthritis resulted in a 50% reduction in joint pain and a 48% reduction in joint stiffness. These results suggest that castor oil is a powerful tool for relieving stiffness and pain in the joints.

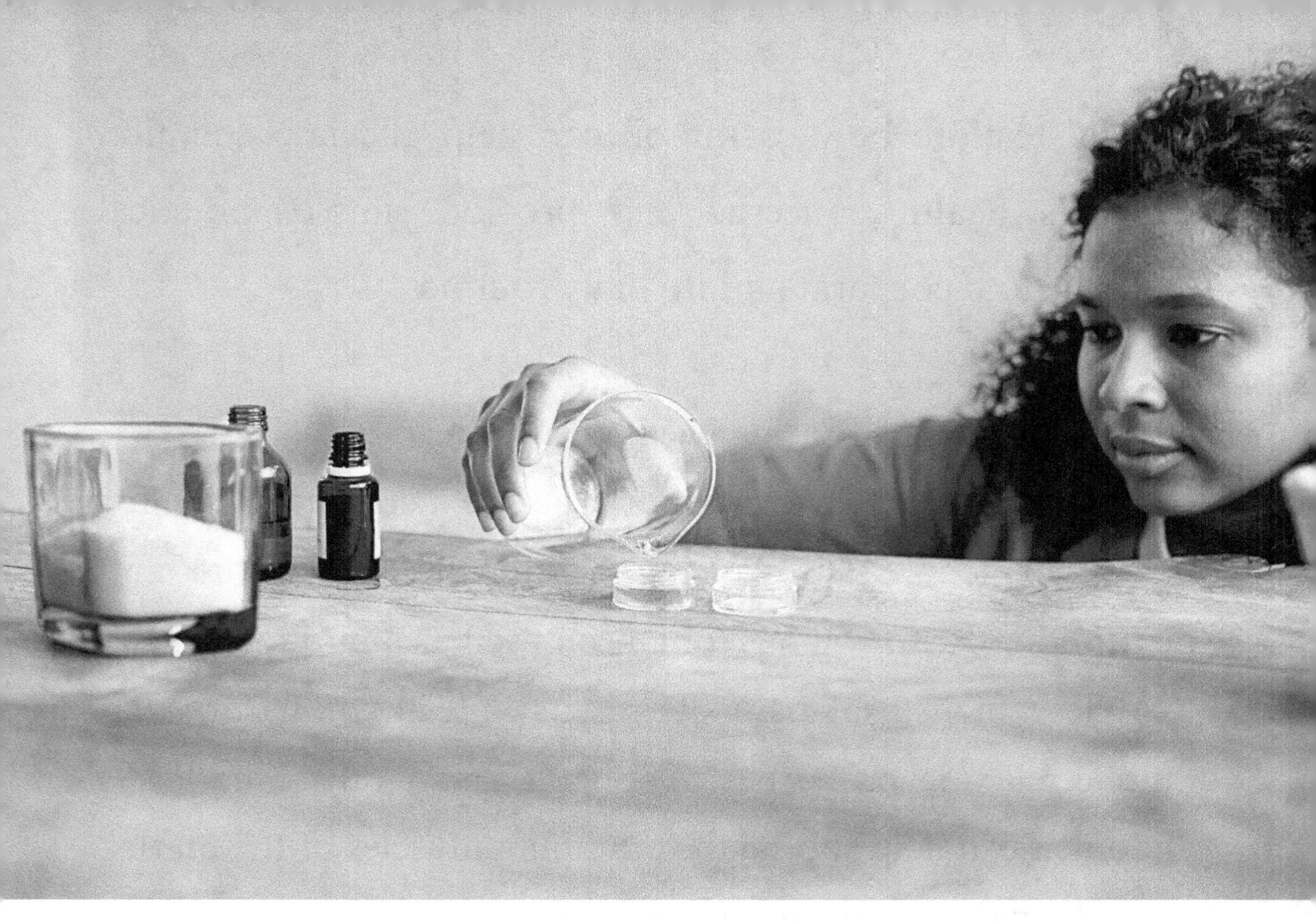

Chapter 6: Castor Oil for Women's Health: Menstrual Relief, Reproductive Wellness, and Postpartum Care

Women have unique health needs, and castor oil has been a valuable tool in addressing many of these needs throughout history. From easing menstrual discomfort to supporting fertility and reproductive health, castor oil's natural properties offer a range of benefits for women of all ages. In this chapter, we will explore how castor oil can help alleviate common women's health concerns and provide simple, practical methods to incorporate it into daily routines.

Easing Menstrual Pain

Menstrual cramps, or dysmenorrhea, are a common issue for many women, often causing significant discomfort and disruption. Castor oil has long been used as a natural remedy to relieve menstrual pain due to its anti-inflammatory and muscle-relaxing properties. Applying castor oil to the lower abdomen can help soothe the cramping muscles of the uterus, reducing pain and promoting relaxation.

NOTE: While some use it for cramps, it may actually increase bleeding. Consult your doctor before using castor oil if you have:

- Any underlying medical conditions
- Are taking medications

Easing Menstrual Pain

Menstrual cramps, or dysmenorrhea, are a common issue for many women, often causing significant discomfort and disruption. Castor oil has long been used as a natural remedy to relieve menstrual pain due to its anti-inflammatory and muscle-relaxing properties. Applying castor oil to the lower abdomen can help soothe the cramping muscles of the uterus, reducing pain and promoting relaxation.

NOTE: While some use it for cramps, it may actually increase bleeding. Consult your doctor before using castor oil if you have:

- Any underlying medical conditions
- Are taking medications

How Castor Oil Helps with Menstrual Cramps:

- Invigorates the Lymphatic System: The lymphatic system is a network of vessels through which toxins and metabolic waste are drained from your vital organs into the surrounding tissues and furthermore moved out into the blood. A healthy lymphatic system is critical for optimal immune function. Castor oil used topically can not only help stimulate lymphatic circulation but has been shown to increase T-cell production in the lymph fluid. T-cells are a particularly important part of your

- immune system, as these cells are directly responsible for killing foreign invaders, like bacteria and viruses. Stimulating proper lymphatic circulation is growing even more important due to our modern, often sedentary lifestyle. We have a variety of essential lymph nodes in our groin that help protect our most vital organs, so stimulating proper circulation is imperative for a high-functioning immune system.

- Supports Liver Function: Our liver is a critical organ that is involved in blood sugar regulation, metabolism and synthesis of fats, storage of vitamins and minerals, and helping us metabolize medications as well as process hormones. The liver is an essential part of optimal hormone balance since it helps regulate estrogen metabolism and can be a major cause of menstrual cramps. Not only is a healthy liver necessary to combat menstrual cramps and endometriosis, but it also helps balance and orchestrate healthy hormone balance necessary for optimal fertility. A castor oil pack over the abdomen can help de-congest the liver to support optimal function and hormonal balance.

- Stimulates the Pelvic Floor: Castor oil is helpful in stimulating healthy venous blood and lymphatic fluid, which helps reduce congestion in the pelvic floor and reduce metabolic waste.

How to Use Castor Oil Packs for cramps

Basically, it's the combination of castor oil and heat that makes this treatment so effective. Heat increases circulation and absorption of the oil into your tissues. Ample time is also essential; get ready to lie down for at least an hour to really let the castor oil do its work.

You can just rub the oil on your belly and cover with an old towel and a heating pad, but the traditional application is much more powerful.

Supplies:

- Organic, cold-pressed castor oil for topical use
- Wool or cotton flannel—approximately 8×30" or so
- A heating pad or hot water bottle
- Gallon ziplock bag or comparable piece of plastic (optional)
- Several old towels

How to:

- Make yourself a comfy spot—on your bed, your couch, or on the floor. You will be there for at least an hour, so make it good—maybe with a pillow for under your knees and another for under your head. Then…

- Cover your comfy spot with old towels (or plastic and old towels) for protection. Reserve one towel to cover yourself with for additional warmth. Castor oil will stain fabrics, so choose your towels carefully and be sure you have enough.! Keep your heating pad and plastic within reach.
- Fold the flannel in thirds, so you have an 8×8 inch square; stitch the open sides together if you're handy like that. This flannel can be used up to 30 times.
- Saturate the flannel with castor oil (pre-warmed if you like).
- Lie down and place the flannel over your lower or upper abdomen (lower for your womb, upper for your liver). Cover this with plastic to protect your heat source (optional). You can use a thin towel if the idea of heated plastic against your body makes you uncomfortable. It will get stained, and it will absorb some of the castor oil intended for your belly, but that's ok.
- Place your heat source on top, cover up, and relax for at least an hour. Heat on your belly is deeply soothing to the nervous system. You can meditate, read, enjoy some mellow music, or nap. This is a time for mental self-care as well as physical.
- After your session, you can rub off any remaining castor oil or massage it into your skin. Drink plenty of water to support the detoxifying effect.

How Often?

The effects of castor oil are cumulative, so it's best to do a few days in a row. I like the rhythm of three days on and the rest of the week off. Do this for a month or more, except as indicated in the cautions below. You can taper off slowly as symptoms improve—maybe down to 3 days in a row once a month, or as part of a seasonal cleanse.

Cautions:

- Do not use castor oil packs during menstruation unless specifically instructed by a knowledgeable healthcare provider.
- Do not use after ovulation if you are trying to conceive. You wouldn't want to move the maybe baby out!
- Do not use castor oil packs on your abdomen if you are pregnant.

Castor Oil Packs for Reproductive Health

Castor oil packs are a traditional remedy used to support reproductive health and balance. These packs are believed to improve blood flow to the uterus and ovaries, support detoxification, and promote lymphatic drainage, making them a gentle yet effective option for various reproductive health concerns.

Benefits of Castor Oil Packs for Women:

Enhances fertility: Castor oil packs are often used by women who are trying to conceive, as they are thought to improve circulation to the reproductive organs and support detoxification, which may help prepare the body for conception.

Supports ovarian health: Regular use of castor oil packs may help with conditions such as ovarian cysts or polycystic ovary syndrome (PCOS) by promoting the natural detoxification of the body and reducing inflammation.

Reduces pelvic congestion: Castor oil packs can help relieve pelvic congestion, a condition that can cause discomfort and pain in the lower abdomen due to poor circulation in the pelvic area.

Shine-Enhancing Hair Serum

Supplies:

- Castor Oil
- Piece of wool or cotton flannel
- Hot water bottle or heating pad

How to:

- Prepare Your Materials: Gather organic castor oil, a piece of wool or cotton flannel, and a hot water bottle or heating pad.

- Soak the Flannel: Saturate the flannel in castor oil until it's well-soaked but not dripping.
- Place the pack: Lie down and place the soaked flannel over your lower abdomen.
- Apply Heat: Put the hot water bottle or heating pad over the flannel, adding a layer of plastic if you wish to protect your clothing and bedding.
- Relax and Rest: Let the pack sit for 45-60 minutes while you relax. You might want to use this time to meditate, read, or practice deep breathing.
- Clean Up: Once done, remove the pack and clean your abdomen. You may save the pack for future use.

When to use:
- Castor oil packs can be applied 3–4 times a week. If trying to conceive, avoid using the packs during menstruation and after ovulation to support the body's natural processes.

Castor Oil for Hormonal Balance

Hormonal imbalances can affect a woman's health in many ways, leading to irregular periods, mood swings, fatigue, and even skin problems. Castor oil's ability to promote detoxification and support the lymphatic system can aid in balancing hormones naturally, making it a helpful addition to any woman's self-care routine.

How Castor Oil Supports Hormonal Health
- **Detoxifies the liver:** The liver plays a key role in hormone regulation by processing and eliminating excess hormones from the body. Castor oil packs applied over the liver can help support its detoxification processes, allowing for better hormonal balance.
- **Stimulates the lymphatic system:** Castor oil promotes lymphatic drainage, which helps the body remove toxins and excess hormones that can contribute to imbalances.

How to use it for hormonal balance:
- Apply a castor oil pack over the liver area (on the right side, just below the rib cage) for 30–60 minutes, 2-3 times a week. This can be particularly beneficial during times of hormonal transition, such as menopause or after discontinuing hormonal contraceptives.

Castor Oil for Menopausal Symptoms

Menopause is a natural phase of life that can bring a range of symptoms, from hot flashes and night sweats to joint pain and mood changes. Castor oil can provide relief from many of these symptoms, thanks to its soothing and balancing effects on the body.

How Castor Oil Eases Menopausal Symptoms

Relieves joint pain: Menopause is often associated with joint stiffness and pain due to declining estrogen levels. Castor oil's anti-inflammatory properties can help soothe sore joints and improve mobility.

Hot flashes: one of the most common symptoms of menopause, can be particularly bothersome. The anti-inflammatory properties of castor oil can help reduce the intensity and frequency of hot flashes when applied topically or used in massage oil. Additionally, massaging the abdomen with castor oil can help alleviate bloating and indigestion, common digestive issues experienced during menopause.

Promotes relaxation: Castor oil's ability to calm the nervous system can help reduce stress and anxiety, which are common during menopause.

Supports hormonal balance: Using castor oil packs over the liver can support detoxification, helping to regulate hormone levels and ease the transition through menopause.

Caster oil for menopause

Supplies:

- Caster Oil
- A (flannel) cloth
- A heating pad or hot water bottle (optional)
- Plastic wrap

- Generously saturate the flannel cloth with castor oil, ensuring it's well-moistened but not dripping.
- Place the cloth on your desired area (often the lower abdomen or liver area) and cover with plastic wrap to prevent leaks.
- Lie down comfortably for 30-60 minutes. Some women find it helpful to place a heating pad set on low over the plastic wrap for added warmth and potential increased absorption.
- Remove the pack and wash the area with warm water. Castor oil can stain, so use an old towel or wear dark clothing to avoid accidents.

Castor Oil for Breast Health

Breast health is an important aspect of overall wellness, and castor oil can be used to support healthy breast tissue. Castor oil packs can help improve lymphatic drainage in the breast area, reduce swelling, and relieve tenderness, making them useful for women dealing with breast discomfort or those looking to promote long-term breast health.

Benefits of Castor Oil for Breast Health:

- **Reduces breast tenderness:** Castor oil's anti-inflammatory properties can help alleviate breast pain or tenderness, especially during menstruation.

- **Improves lymphatic flow:** One of the main processes occurring in our breast tissue is lymphatic flow. Lymphatic flow slows down in various bodily parts when stress and inflammation are applied, which leads to obstructions. Tight bras, bras composed of plastic or materials that disturb hormones, and environmental stressors are some of the major factors influencing lymphatic flow within breast tissue. Easy techniques like wearing castor oil, exercising the upper body, and diaphragmatic breathing can help enhance lymphatic circulation, which aids in the removal of toxins.

- **Stimulating Smooth Muscle:** Organs and blood vessels, especially the lymphatic system, contain smooth muscle. This kind of muscle plays a critical role in hormone balance and general health by aiding in tissue detoxification. Smooth muscle efficacy decreases when these tissues are impacted by stress and inflammation. A holistic approach to detoxifying those body parts and stimulating smooth muscle, particularly in breast tissue, is through the use of castor oil, which also lowers the likelihood of developing new health issues.

- **Supports detoxification:** Because castor oil stimulates the lymphatic system, it may aid the body in getting rid of toxins that build up in breast tissue.

- Castor oil
- 3 hand towels or 3 bath towels (Depending on the size of your breasts)
- piece of plastic (garbage bag will do)
- Heavy blanket to hold the heat in
- Something to heat 2 of the towels (Large turkey roaster, oven or microwave)
- Place to sit or lay down that is covered to prevent water seepage during the process.

- Wet 2 towels, wring out by hand, and heat them.
- Wet the third towel with cold tap water and wring out. (Usually not necessary to put it in the fridge to cool it more, but you want it cold.).
- Rub a thin layer of castor oil into the axillary (armpits) and over the entire breasts. Most breast lymph drains into the axillary nodes, making it critical to have this area flowing.
- Apply hot towel wrapping to cover the armpits and breasts. Be sure it is hot enough to be therapeutic but not burn your skin.

- Cover with plastic and heavy blanket to hold the heat in.
- Allow to sit for 5-10 min. or until the towel begins to cool down.
- Apply the second hot towel to the skin and put the first hot towel over top of the fresh one to further keep the heat in. Cover again and let sit until the towel begins to cool down.
- Remove the hot towels and apply the cold one (breathe!) pressing the cold towel into the axillary especially. Do NOT skip this step! This is necessary to flush the area. Without this step, you will feel congested and not well. It warms up quickly, just shocking at first. **KEEP THIS ON UNTIL YOUR BODY HEATS THE COLD TOWEL**, usually 5-10 min.

NOTE: If you have cancer, please consult your physician before using this method of self-treatment.

Inducing Labor with Castor Oil

Castor oil has long been used as a traditional remedy to induce labor naturally. While its effectiveness and safety remain topics of debate among medical professionals, many women have turned to castor oil to stimulate contractions when they are past their due date or facing a slow labor progression. However, never try any home remedies to induce labor without speaking with your medical professional first. It can be difficult to wait for a baby's much-anticipated arrival, but induced labor too early or using questionable methods isn't safe.

Is Caster Oil Safe for Inducing Labor?

To consider the overall safety of castor oil for inducing labor, it will be good to take a look at the individual ingredients involved in the recipe;

Castor Oil: One of castor oil's most common uses is as a laxative. This is because castor oil can cause little spasms in the intestines. Similarly, it can cause spasming of the uterine muscles, which can lead to contractions and Induce labor. But consuming castor oil can also lead to severe diarrhea, nausea, and vomiting. In a word, it's unpleasant. It's very important to watch out for dehydration if taking castor oil. Additionally, castor oil may cause contractions that stay irregular or become extremely painful. This can cause exhaustion or additional stress on mom and baby. This is one reason why castor oil shouldn't be used during pregnancy without a healthcare professional's guidance and supervision.

Lemon verbena oil: There isn't a lot of research around the use of lemon verbena oil in pregnancy and labor. Speak with your midwife about their views on you ingesting it.

Almond butter: If you have a nut allergy, this is certainly an ingredient to be aware of. But for others, it's generally safe. If you have an almond allergy, it may be possible to substitute another type of nut butter. Speak to your doctor or midwife about another ingredient that can replace this.

Apricot juice: Apricot juice is a great source of vitamins and minerals. Unless you have a specific allergy to apricots, it's probably safe to consume apricots throughout your pregnancy. (Though, like everything, consumption in moderation is key!)

How to Use Castor Oil for Labor Induction

Castor oil is the labor-inducing ingredient, while the others are there primarily to mask the taste of. Castor oil, and these combinations are usually called Midwives Brew.

Classic Midwives Brew Recipe

- 2 tablespoons of almond butter
- 1 cup of apricot juice
- 2 tablespoons of castor oil
- 1 cup of lemon verbena tea (room temperature)

- Brew the lemon verbena tea and let it cool to room temperature.
- Blend the apricot juice, almond butter, castor oil, and tea together until smooth.
- Drink the mixture on an empty stomach for best results, ideally in the early morning.

Different Recipes for Midwives Brew

Midwives Brew with Pineapple Juice

- 1 cup of pineapple juice (instead of apricot juice)
- 2 tablespoons of almond butter
- 2 tablespoons of castor oil
- 1 cup of lemon verbena tea (room temperature)

- Brew the lemon verbena tea and let it cool to room temperature.
- Blend the pineapple juice, almond butter, castor oil, and tea together until smooth.
- Drink the mixture on an empty stomach for best results, ideally in the early morning.

Midwives Brew with Peanut Butter

Supplies:

- 2 tablespoons of peanut butter (instead of almond butter)
- 1 cup of apricot juice
- 2 tablespoons of castor oil
- 1 cup of lemon verbena tea (room temperature)

How to:

- Brew the lemon verbena tea and let it cool to room temperature.
- Blend the apricot juice, peanut butter, castor oil, and tea together until smooth.
- Drink the mixture on an empty stomach for best results, ideally in the early morning.

Midwives Brew with Herbal Tea Variation

- 1 cup of herbal tea (such as red raspberry leaf tea) instead of lemon verbena tea
- 2 tablespoons of almond butter
- 1 cup of apricot juice
- 2 tablespoons of castor oil

- Brew the herbal tea and let it cool to room temperature.
- Blend the apricot juice, almond butter, castor oil, and tea together until smooth.
- Drink the mixture on an empty stomach for best results, ideally in the early morning.

Midwives Brew with Essential Oils

- 1 drop of essential oil (such as clary sage) added to the mixture
- 2 tablespoons of almond butter
- 1 cup of apricot juice
- 2 tablespoons of castor oil
- 1 cup of lemon verbena tea (room temperature)

- Brew the lemon verbena tea and let it cool to room temperature.
- Blend the apricot juice, almond butter, castor oil, and tea together until smooth.
- Add 1 drop of essential oil to the mixture.
- Drink the mixture on an empty stomach for best results, ideally in the early morning.

Effectiveness of Castor Oil in Inducing Labor

Although there are a lot of anecdotal reports on the success of Caster oil, there's a lack of research behind it. Looking at the scientific effectiveness of castor oil, there aren't a lot of studies on it, and the results vary. These are some studies made by the National Library of Medicine, U.S.A.:

- In one of their older studies, of 103 women who were at least 40 weeks pregnant, half were given castor oil and half had no treatment. Of those given castor oil, nearly 60 percent were in active labor within 24 hours. (And for those who had castor oil-induced labor, more than 80 percent gave birth vaginally.)

- Another study published in 2009, gave a less enthusiastic finding for castor oil. It suggested the oil's effects are neither particularly helpful nor harmful in inducing labors.

- And a review noted the effectiveness of castor oil for inducing labor but cautioned that the quality of the studies may make results questionable. Also of note: Researchers found that all women who took castor oil felt nauseous. So, for the time being, the formal scientific jury still appears to be out. Basically, more research is needed, especially when it comes to the ingredients other than castor oil, but for castor oil, too.

NOTE: It's also worth noting that castor oil should only be used after 40 weeks of pregnancy or under the advice of your healthcare provider. Additionally, an induction is more likely to be successful when the body is already ready to go into labor.

Possible Side Effects

Though castor oil can help induce labor, it comes with a variety of potential side effects.

- **Nausea and Vomiting:** Castor oil's strong laxative properties often lead to nausea and vomiting, making it unpleasant for many women.

- **Diarrhea and Dehydration:** Since castor oil stimulates the bowels, it can cause diarrhea, leading to dehydration. Staying hydrated is crucial if you choose this method.

- **Uterine Hyperstimulation:** There is a risk of hyperstimulation, where the uterus contracts too frequently or strongly. This can reduce blood flow to the baby and cause distress, making it a risky option for some women.

- **Fatigue:** The combination of bowel movements and potential dehydration can leave the body fatigued, which may be counterproductive during labor.

Alternatives to Castor Oil for Inducing Labor

If castor oil seems too risky or unappealing, there are other natural ways to encourage labor, such as:

- **Walking:** Light exercise like walking may help position the baby better and encourage contractions.

- Sex: Intercourse may help trigger labor due to the presence of prostaglandins in semen.

- Acupuncture or Acupressure: These alternative therapies are believed by some to stimulate labor.

- Nipple Stimulation: This method can trigger the release of oxytocin, which can lead to contractions.

Castor Oil for Postpartum Care

The postpartum period can be challenging as the body recovers from childbirth. Castor oil's healing and restorative properties make it a valuable tool for supporting postpartum recovery. From relieving sore muscles to promoting wound healing, castor oil can help new mothers feel more comfortable during this time.

Here's how castor oil packs can help your postpartum recovery:

- **Womb and abdomen:** A gentle pack over this area nourishes your recovering womb and supports a smooth return of your digestive system. This could potentially reduce postpartum uterine swelling and offer some relief from cramping.

- **Breasts:** If you experience blocked milk ducts or mastitis, the warmth of a castor oil pack can bring welcome relief. Follow with a gentle massage to help with milk flow. Be sure to wipe your nipple afterward and continue to breastfeed your baby frequently.

- **C-section scars:** Once your incision is fully healed, castor oil packs can be an incredible support for C-section and perineal tears. They help soften scar tissue, minimizing any long-term tightness or discomfort. Combine them with gentle scar massage for the best results.

- **Stress Reduction & Self-Care:** Taking time to apply a castor oil pack can be a relaxing self-care ritual, promoting much-needed calmness during the hectic postpartum period.

How to:

- For muscle soreness, massage castor oil into the affected areas daily.
- For scar healing, gently apply castor oil to the scarred area once the wound has fully closed. Continue use until the scar softens and fades.

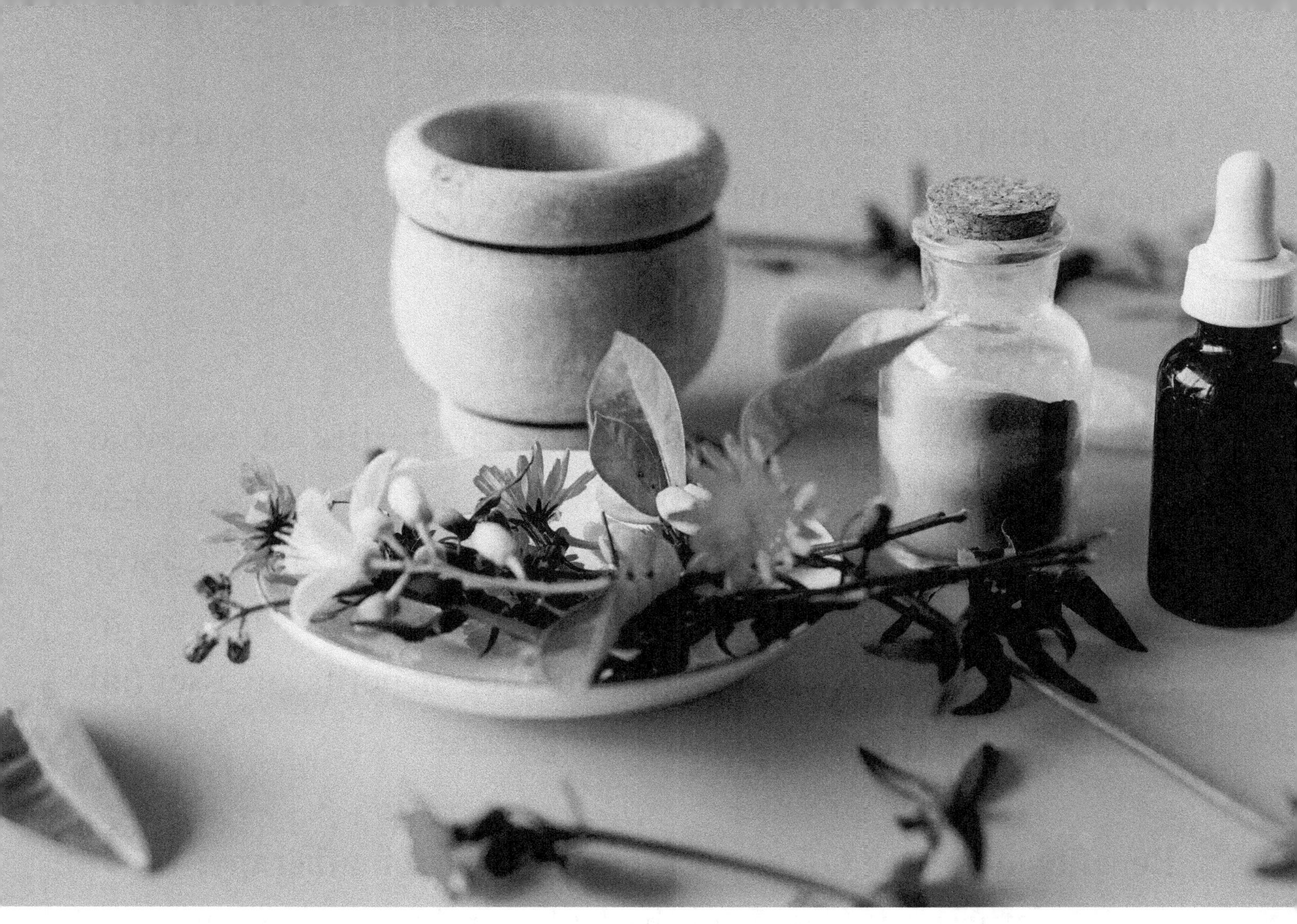

Chapter 7: Aromatherapy and Emotional Well-being: Stress Relief and Healing with Castor Oil

Aromatherapy is a powerful method of using essential oils and natural extracts to promote emotional and physical well-being. While castor oil is not typically recognized for its aromatic qualities, it plays a vital role as a carrier oil in aromatherapy. It is an excellent base for mixing essential oils, and its moisturizing, soothing properties enhance the therapeutic effects of aromatherapy.

In this chapter, we will explore how castor oil can be used in aromatherapy to support emotional well-being, relieve stress, and enhance massage therapy experiences.

Castor Oil in Aromatherapy

Aromatherapy relies on the healing properties of essential oils extracted from plants, but these concentrated oils often need to be diluted in a carrier oil for safe application. Castor oil, with its thick consistency and neutral scent, makes an excellent carrier oil that can extend the benefits of essential oils without overpowering their fragrance.

Benefits of Castor Oil as a Carrier Oil in Aromatherapy:

- Moisturizing: Castor oil hydrates and nourishes the skin, enhancing the overall experience of aromatherapy. It helps keep the skin supple and protected from dryness.
- Absorption: While castor oil is thicker than many other carrier oils, it penetrates deep into the skin, allowing the essential oils to be absorbed effectively and prolonging their benefits.
- Neutral Scent: Castor oil has a mild scent that doesn't interfere with the aroma of essential oils, making it an ideal base for aromatic blends.

How Castor Oil Supports Emotional Well-being:

- **Stress Relief:** When combined with essential oils known for their calming properties (such as lavender, chamomile, or frankincense), castor oil helps deliver a grounding and relaxing effect.
- **Enhancing Mood:** The gentle warmth of castor oil, when massaged into the skin or used in a compress, helps release muscle tension and promotes relaxation, aiding in emotional release and mood enhancement.

Calming Blend for Stress Relief

Castor oil can be combined with essential oils to create a soothing blend that promotes relaxation, reduces anxiety, and helps relieve stress. This blend can be used during massages, applied to pulse points, or simply inhaled for its calming effects.

Supplies:

- 2 tablespoons of castor oil
- 5 drops of lavender essential oil (for calming)
- 3 drops of chamomile essential oil (for relaxation)
- 2 drops of frankincense essential oil (for grounding)

- In a small bowl or bottle, combine the castor oil with the essential oils.
- Gently stir or shake the mixture to ensure the oils are well-blended.
- For a relaxing massage: Apply the mixture to the back, shoulders, neck, or any area where tension is held. Massage gently to help release tension and promote relaxation.
- For stress relief on the go: Dab a small amount of the blend onto your wrists or temples. Inhale deeply to benefit from the calming aroma.
- For an aromatic bath: Add the oil blend to a warm bath to relax both the mind and body after a stressful day.

Why This Blend Works:

Lavender essential oil is well-known for its ability to calm the nervous system, reduce anxiety, and promote better sleep.

Chamomile essential oil adds a soothing, anti-inflammatory effect that helps relax muscles and ease emotional stress.

Frankincense essential oil is often used in meditation for its grounding properties. It can help clear the mind, reduce feelings of overwhelm, and promote a sense of peace.

Together with castor oil, these essential oils work synergistically to deliver deep relaxation and emotional relief.

Castor Oil for Massage Therapy

Massage therapy is a time-honored practice that promotes both physical and emotional well-being. Using castor oil in massage therapy can enhance the experience by offering deep moisture and helping the essential oils penetrate more effectively into the skin.

Why Castor Oil is Effective for Massage:
- **Deep Moisturization:** Castor oil's thick, emollient nature makes it ideal for massages. It deeply hydrates the skin, making it smooth and nourished after the treatment.
- **Pain Relief**: Castor oil has anti-inflammatory properties that can help relieve sore muscles and reduce joint pain during a massage. Its warming effect can also promote circulation, aiding in pain relief.
- **Long-Lasting Effect**: Due to its slow absorption rate, castor oil allows for longer massages without the need to frequently reapply, which is particularly useful for deep tissue and therapeutic massages.

Emotional Benefits of Castor Oil Massage:
- Relaxation and Stress Reduction: Massage with castor oil helps to calm the nervous system, releasing both physical and emotional tension. This process can bring about feelings of relaxation, reduce stress, and promote emotional balance.

- **Enhanced Sleep:** Regular castor oil massages, especially when combined with calming essential oils, can help improve sleep quality by reducing stress and promoting relaxation.
- **Mood Enhancement:** By releasing stored tension in the body, a castor oil massage can enhance mood and emotional well-being, making it a powerful tool in emotional self-care.

Supplies:

- Caster oil
- Lavender oil, peppermint

How to:

- **Prepare the oil blend:** Warm a small amount of castor oil in your hands or a bowl. If desired, add a few drops of essential oils such as lavender, eucalyptus, or peppermint for additional relaxation or pain relief.
- **Apply to the body:** Gently apply the oil to the desired areas (back, shoulders, legs, etc.), using firm but gentle strokes to massage it into the skin.
- **Focus on tension points:** Pay special attention to areas where tension tends to accumulate, such as the neck, shoulders, and lower back. The thickness of the castor oil helps facilitate deeper massage techniques.

- **Relax and breathe deeply:** Allow yourself or the person receiving the massage to breathe deeply and relax during the session. The oil's soothing warmth, combined with the scent of essential oils, can help release emotional stress and promote a calming atmosphere.
- **Post-massage care:** After the massage, leave the oil on the skin for 15–30 minutes to allow full absorption. If needed, gently wipe off excess oil with a warm towel or take a warm shower.

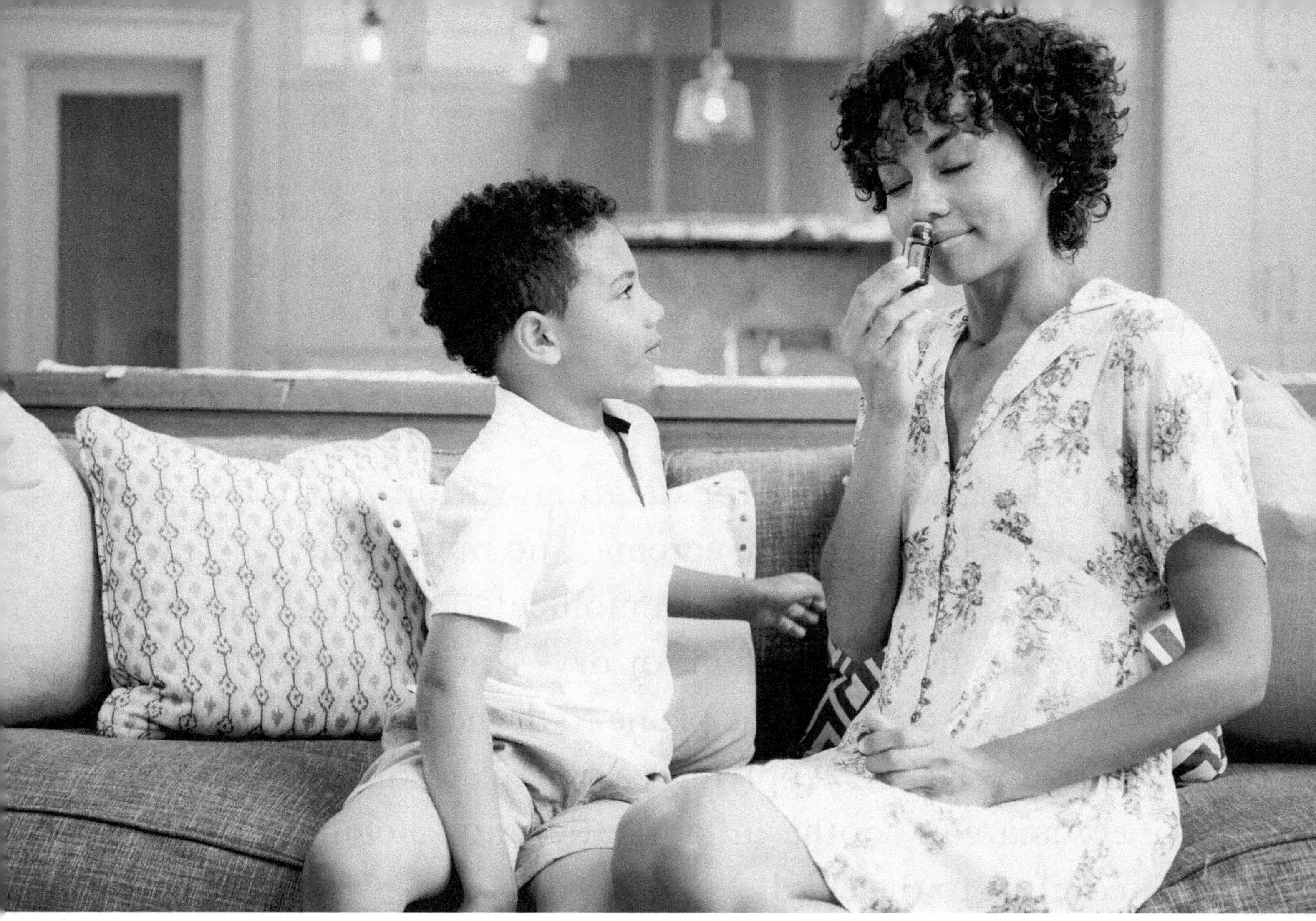

Chapter 8: Castor Oil for Children's Health and Pet Care: Safe Applications and Benefits

Castor oil is a versatile natural remedy that can be a valuable addition to a family's wellness toolkit. Its gentle nature and broad range of uses make it particularly suitable for children's health. From addressing minor ailments to supporting overall well-being, castor oil offers various safe and effective applications for children. This chapter will explore the safe uses of castor oil for children, how it can help treat common childhood ailments, and even its application in pet care.

Safe Uses for Children

While castor oil is generally safe for topical use on children, it's essential to follow specific guidelines to ensure its safe application.

1. Skin Care

Castor oil is excellent for treating various skin issues in children, such as dry skin, eczema, and minor cuts.

- Moisturizing: Due to its emollient properties, castor oil provides deep hydration for dry, sensitive skin, making it ideal for treating areas prone to dryness.
- Eczema Relief: Applying castor oil to areas affected by eczema can soothe inflammation and itching, providing comfort to the child.
- Minor Cuts and Scrapes: Castor oil's antibacterial properties can help prevent infections in minor cuts, while its moisturizing effect supports healing.

2. Digestive Health

Constipation and digestive discomfort are common among children. Castor oil can help address these issues when used appropriately.

- External Application for Constipation: A gentle abdominal massage with warmed castor oil can stimulate bowel movements without the need for internal ingestion, making it a safer option for children.

- Gas Relief: Massaging castor oil onto the abdomen can help relieve gas and colicky pain in infants and young children.

3. Hair Care

Castor oil is beneficial for children's hair and scalp, promoting healthy growth and addressing common scalp issues.

- Moisturizing the Scalp: Regular application can help prevent dryness and flakiness.
- Promoting Healthy Hair Growth: The nutrients in castor oil nourish the hair follicles, potentially supporting stronger and healthier hair.
-

Treating Childhood Ailments

Castor oil can serve as a natural remedy for several common childhood ailments. Its anti-inflammatory and soothing properties make it an excellent choice for addressing various health concerns.

1. Diaper Rash

Diaper rash is a frequent issue for infants and toddlers. Castor oil can effectively soothe and heal irritated skin.

- How to Use: After changing a diaper, apply a thin layer of castor oil to the affected area to protect and heal the skin.

NOTE: Be careful to avoid application on or around areas such as the baby's lips, nose, eyes, and genitals.

- Avoid application on broken skin, as it can also irritate your baby's skin.
- Consult with your doctor to understand what category of Castor oil is suitable for your baby—cold-pressed, processed, etc.
- Make sure that your baby does not ingest the oil.

2. Cough and Congestion

When children have colds or respiratory issues, castor oil can be beneficial when used topically. Castor oil rubs are a great way to bring comfort to someone experiencing a cold, and bring down any inflammation. Castor oil can be applied to the chest, neck, and face, and heat can be applied by a hot water bottle to the chest over top to help bring some comfort during the cold.

- **How to Use**: A warm castor oil massage on the chest can help relieve congestion and ease coughing. It's best combined with a few drops of eucalyptus or peppermint essential oil for added respiratory benefits.

3. Earaches

While castor oil cannot cure ear infections, it can provide relief from the pain associated with earaches.

- **How to Use**: Gently massage warmed castor oil around the outer ear to reduce pain and inflammation. Note: Avoid placing oil directly in the ear canal.

4. Fever and Pain Relief

Castor oil helps reduce fever and headaches in childhood by exerting anti-inflammatory and analgesic effects. When applied topically to the skin, it can penetrate deeply and alleviate inflammation, thus reducing fever-related discomfort. Additionally, massaging the oil onto the temples or forehead can help ease headache pain by promoting relaxation and improving blood circulation in the affected areas.

- **How to Use:** Apply a warm castor oil pack to the abdomen or back to relieve discomfort associated with fever or body aches.

Pet Care

Castor oil is not only beneficial for children; it can also be safely used for pet care. Many pets can benefit from the soothing and moisturizing properties of castor oil, making it a helpful addition to their health regimen.

How to Safely Apply Castor Oil to Your Dog's Skin

Patch Testing: Prior to widespread use, perform a patch test by applying a small amount of diluted castor oil to a small area of your dog's skin. Monitor for any adverse reactions, such as redness or itching.

Dilution Ratios: Always dilute castor oil before applying it to your dog's skin. Mix it with a carrier oil like coconut oil in a 1:1 ratio. This ensures a safe and effective application.

Massage Techniques: Gently massage the diluted castor oil into your dog's skin. This not only aids in absorption but also creates a bonding experience between you and your pet.

Incorporating Castor Oil into Your Dog's Diet

Mixing with Food: If you choose to add castor oil to your dog's diet, we recommend 100% pure organic caster oil. Start with small amounts and mix it into their food to make ingestion more palatable. Monitor your dog's response and adjust the quantity as needed.

Dosage Guidelines: Consult your veterinarian to determine the appropriate dosage for your dog's size, breed, and health status. Too much castor oil can lead to digestive issues, so it's crucial to follow professional advice.

2. Flea and Tick Prevention

While castor oil is not a substitute for veterinary treatments, it can serve as a supplementary deterrent against fleas and ticks.

- **How to Use**: Mix castor oil with water and a few drops of essential oils (like lavender or cedarwood) to create a natural spray. Apply it lightly to your pet's fur, avoiding the face and eyes.

3. Moisturizing Paw Pads

Pets' paw pads can become dry and cracked, especially in winter. Castor oil can help keep them soft and healthy.

- **How to Use:** Massage a small amount of castor oil into your pet's paw pads to keep them moisturized and protected.

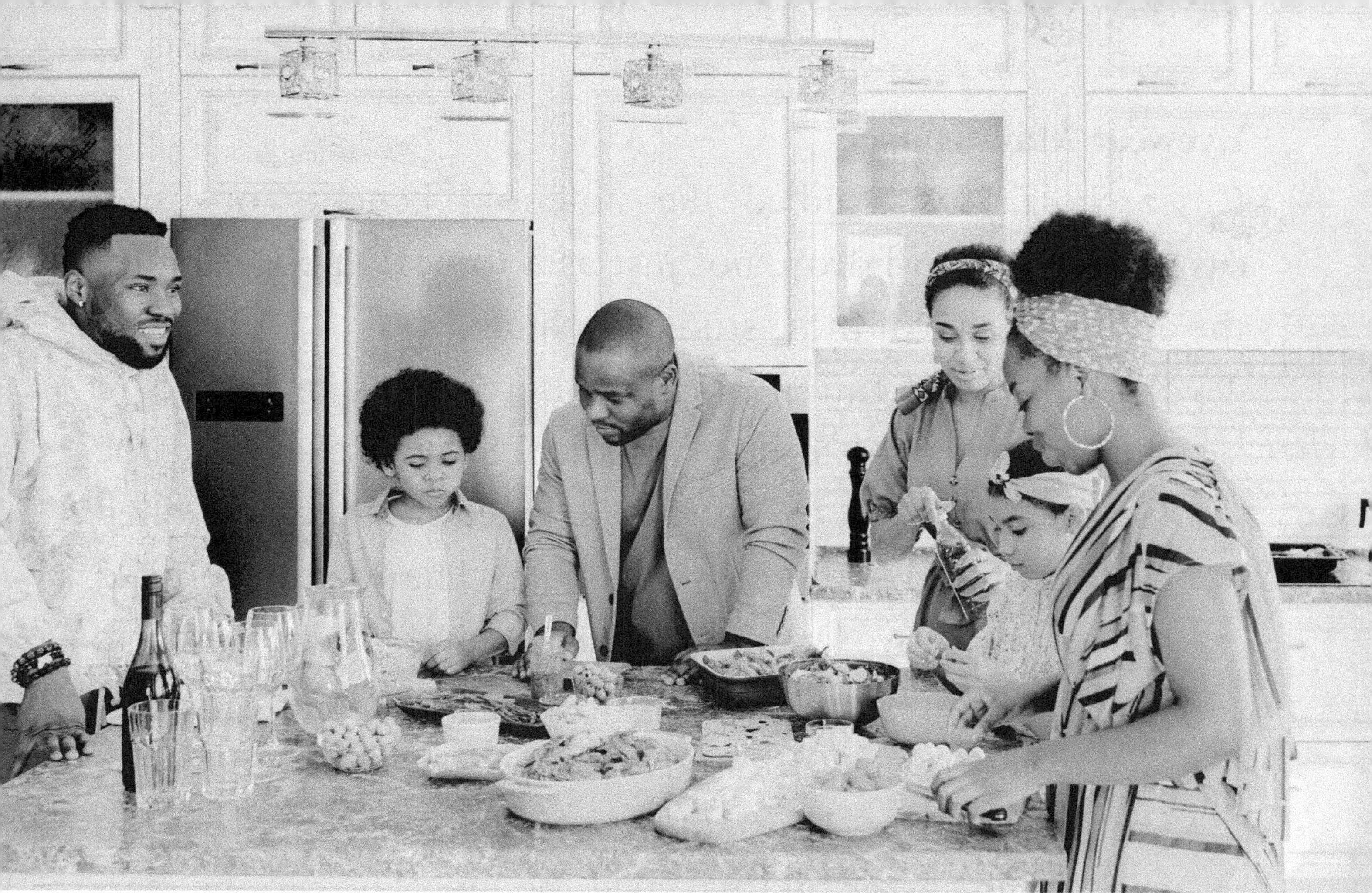

Chapter 9: Versatile Household Uses of Castor Oil: From Personal Care to Home Maintenance

Castor oil is not just a natural remedy for health and wellness; it also has numerous household uses that make it a versatile product to keep around. From personal care to maintaining everyday items, castor oil's moisturizing and protective properties provide easy, natural solutions. In this chapter, we will explore some of the lesser-known, yet highly useful, ways castor oil can be employed around the home, including eyewear maintenance, lip care, nail and cuticle treatment, sunburn relief, and even leather conditioning.

Eyewear Maintenance

Researchers have studied the potential benefits of using castor oil as an eye drop, not just as a topical application on the eyelids. Some of these studies include:

- A 2014 investigation on animals that was published in the Journal of Veterinary Medical Science examined the treatment of pig eyes using a solution that contained castor oil and sodium hyaluronate. The mixture proved to be protective against dry eyes, and the researchers suggested applying the mixture as a substitute for tears.

- According to a 2010 study that was written up in the journal Contact Lens and Anterior Eye, an eye drop containing castor oil thickened the lipid layer in the tear, which helped to relieve dry eyes.

- The use of castor oil-containing eye drops in the treatment of meibomian gland dysfunction (MGD), a frequent cause of dry eye, was examined in a 2002 study that was published in the journal Ophthalmology. Participants in the study applied a mixture of 5 percent polyoxyethylene castor oil and 2 percent castor oil. The study participants did not report any unfavorable side effects, and the researchers discovered that the castor oil eye drops were successful in treating MGD.

The Advantages of Eye Drops with Castor Oil

A multipurpose substance, castor oil may be beneficial for conditions such as meibomian gland dysfunction (MGD). This disorder is a prevalent cause of dry eyes. MGD has been demonstrated to respond well to a modest concentration of castor oil eye drops. They enhance the lipids and tears' stability in your eyes. The drops maintain the health of your eyes by thickening the lipid layer, avoiding infection, and relieving symptoms.

Castor oil-containing eye drops also aid in the relief of dry eye symptoms. Your eyes may get dryer, more itchy, and more painful as a result of the oil's reduction of tear evaporation. It also aids in general dryness because of its capacity to regulate tear production.

Castor has therapeutic qualities because of its antibacterial and anti-inflammatory qualities. Castor oil is harmless for your eyes and helps to increase the lipids in your tear film.

The duration of castor oil eye drops is another advantage. They could remain in your eyes for up to four hours, according to studies.

Tips for Using Castor Oil Eye Drops

It might be challenging to use eye drops for the first time, particularly if you're not used to putting items in your eyes. Wash your hands first, and make sure a fresh towel is close at hand. Then:

- Tilt your head back and place your index finger on the soft spot below your lower lid. Gently pull down.
- Look up at the ceiling and squeeze one drop into the pouch formed in your lower lid.
- Don't wipe your eye. Close it and let the eye drop spread out. This will make sure that the drops have been absorbed.

Note: If you notice side effects like blurry vision, itchiness, or swelling, you may be having an allergic reaction. Other symptoms include:
- Trouble breathing
- Dizziness
- Nausea

Stop using the eye drops right away and call your doctor. Without treatment, a reaction could cause complications with your eyes and eyesight.

Lip Care

Castor oil is a fantastic natural moisturizer that can help keep your lips soft, smooth, and hydrated, especially in dry or cold weather.

- **Moisturizing Dry Lips:** The fatty acids in castor oil deeply moisturize and lock in hydration, making it a great remedy for chapped or dry lips. It helps create a protective barrier that keeps lips hydrated for longer.
- **How to Use:** Apply a small amount of castor oil directly to your lips using your finger or a cotton swab. For added benefits, you can mix castor oil with a drop of honey or coconut oil to create a soothing lip balm.
- **Bonus Tip:** If you have severely chapped lips, applying castor oil before bed and leaving it on overnight can speed up the healing process.

Nail and Cuticle Care

Suffering with brittle and dry nails? Want to grow your nails longer but are unable to do so because you're scared they'll break? Castor oil is an all-in-one treatment that may help your brittle nails grow and strengthen them. The health of your nails may be improved with the use of castor oil. In addition to this, it maintains the nails as well as nourishes and moisturizes them in order to improve nail strength.

- **Strengthening Nails:** Castor oil is rich in vitamin E and essential fatty acids, which help strengthen weak or brittle nails. Regular use can prevent breakage and encourage nail growth.
- **Moisturizing Cuticles:** Castor oil's hydrating properties help soften dry and cracked cuticles, which can prevent hangnails and other issues associated with poorly maintained cuticles.

Upkeep Nail Health with Castor Oil and Olive Oil

Supplies:

- 15 drops of castor oil
- 15 drops of extra virgin olive oil
- Tea tree essential oil or thyme essential oil (optional)

How to:

- The nails need to be manicured and the nail polish removed. Use a nail polish remover to remove the nail polish. Use a cutter and file to cut long nails and get them to shape.
- Next, wash and scrub the fingers to remove dead skin.
- Mix the oils and use a cotton pad to soak the oil. Now, apply the pad to the cuticles of the nails.
- Massage the oil on the nails and fingertips with the cotton pad for a few minutes. Leave it overnight.

For Preventing Hand Infections

- 1 tablespoon of castor oil,
- 1 tablespoon of coconut oil, and
- 1½ teaspoon of honey.

- Mix the ingredients well until you get a thick paste.
- Apply this paste to your nails twice a day before sleeping and in the morning as well. And in the evening as well.
- Cover the nails with cotton or gauze for at least one hour before going to bed. You can also do it overnight by applying castor oil before you go to sleep and then removing it after washing up at least 30 minutes later.
- This will help your nails to be stronger and healthier than they are now. This is for both left hand and right hand, depending on which one you are used to using more often.

Castor Oil for Oral Health

Castor oil, widely known for its skincare and wellness benefits, also plays a significant role in promoting oral health. Thanks to its anti-inflammatory, antimicrobial, and moisturizing properties, castor oil can be a natural solution for maintaining a clean and healthy mouth. This ancient remedy can assist in preventing oral issues such as bad breath, gum disease, and even tooth decay. Let's explore how castor oil can be incorporated into your oral hygiene routine.

1. Antibacterial and Antifungal Properties

The mouth is home to a multitude of bacteria, both good and bad. When harmful bacteria accumulate, they can lead to various oral health issues, including gum disease and cavities. Castor oil contains ricinoleic acid, which has potent antibacterial and antifungal properties, helping to reduce harmful bacteria in the mouth.

- Why It Works: Castor oil can fight common oral pathogens such as Candida albicans, a fungus that causes oral thrush, and Streptococcus mutans, a bacterium responsible for tooth decay. By eliminating these harmful microbes, castor oil helps maintain a healthy balance of bacteria in the mouth, preventing infections and promoting overall oral health.

2. Reducing Gum Inflammation and Treating Gingivitis

Gum inflammation, or gingivitis, is a common condition that affects many people and can lead to more severe forms of gum disease if left untreated. Symptoms include redness, swelling, and bleeding of the gums, often caused by bacterial plaque buildup. Castor oil's anti-inflammatory properties make it an effective treatment for reducing gum inflammation.

How to Use: Apply a small amount of castor oil to inflamed or irritated gums using a clean cotton swab or your fingertip. Gently massage it into the gums to reduce swelling and pain. The ricinoleic acid in castor oil helps soothe the inflamed tissue while fighting the bacteria that cause gingivitis.

3. Healing Mouth Sores and Oral Infections

Mouth sores, including canker sores and cold sores, can be painful and slow to heal. Castor oil, with its antimicrobial and soothing effects, can speed up the healing process and provide relief from discomfort.

Why It Works: Castor oil forms a protective barrier over the sore, helping it heal faster while keeping bacteria at bay. Its moisturizing properties also prevent the sore from drying out, which can exacerbate pain.

How to Use: Apply a drop of castor oil directly to the sore several times a day. For canker sores, use a cotton swab to apply the oil gently. Repeat the process until the sore heals completely.

4. Treating Dry Mouth

Dry mouth, or xerostomia, is a condition in which the salivary glands in the mouth do not produce enough saliva. This can lead to discomfort, difficulty in swallowing, bad breath, and an increased risk of cavities. Castor oil can help alleviate the symptoms of dry mouth by providing moisture and promoting saliva production.

- **How to Use**: Swish a small amount of castor oil in your mouth for 1-2 minutes, then spit it out. The oil will coat the oral tissues and help relieve dryness, making it an effective natural remedy for those suffering from dry mouth. You can also rub a small amount of castor oil on the tongue and gums before bed to keep the mouth moist overnight.

5. Freshening Breath

Bad breath, or halitosis, is often caused by bacteria buildup in the mouth. Castor oil's antimicrobial properties can help combat these bacteria, leaving your mouth feeling fresh and clean.

- How to Use: Add a drop of castor oil to your toothpaste or use it as part of an oil-pulling routine (see below) to freshen your breath. The oil's ability to eliminate odor-causing bacteria will leave your mouth smelling and feeling fresher for longer.

6. Oil Pulling with Castor Oil

One of the most popular methods of using castor oil for oral health is through a practice called oil pulling. Oil pulling is an ancient Ayurvedic practice that involves swishing oil in your mouth to "pull" toxins out, whiten teeth, and promote oral hygiene.

- **How It Works**: Swishing castor oil around your mouth helps dislodge plaque and bacteria, reduces bad breath, and promotes gum health. It also helps remove toxins from the body, leading to a cleaner and healthier oral cavity.
- **How to Oil Pull**:
  a. Take 1 tablespoon of castor oil and swish it around in your mouth for 10-15 minutes.
  b. Be sure to swish it gently, allowing the oil to reach all areas of your mouth.
  c. Spit the oil out (never swallow it, as it contains toxins and bacteria), then rinse your mouth with warm water.
  d. Brush your teeth afterward to remove any residue.

Performing oil pulling regularly can help maintain oral health and keep your teeth and gums in top condition.

7. Preventing Tooth Decay

Due to its antibacterial properties, castor oil can help prevent **tooth decay** by reducing harmful bacteria in the mouth. Plaque, the sticky substance that forms on teeth, is often the result of bacterial accumulation and can lead to cavities if not properly managed.

- **How to Use**: As a preventive measure, you can add a few drops of castor oil to your toothbrush or mix it with your regular toothpaste when brushing your teeth. This helps reduce plaque formation and keeps harmful bacteria under control.

Leather Conditioner

Leather items, such as shoes, bags, jackets, or furniture, can dry out and crack over time if not properly maintained. Castor oil serves as an excellent natural leather conditioner, helping to preserve and protect leather goods. High-quality leather conditioner and polish can be easily purchased, but if you're up for a homemade adventure, give this DIY leather conditioner a try.

- 1/2 cup castor oil
- 2 tablespoons shea or coconut butter
- 1/2 cup sweet almond oil
- 2 tablespoons beeswax

- Melt butter and beeswax in a medium saucepan over medium-low heat, stirring constantly to avoid burning or boiling.
- Keep stirring, and add the sweet almond oil
- After almond oil is fully blended, add castor oil. Stir until castor oil is well blended, and continue to heat for 4-5 minutes, but do not allow to boil.
- Pour mixture into empty tins, filling to about a quarter from the top, and allow to cool.
- You can adjust the ratio of your leather conditioner recipe depending on how firm you want your conditioner. More beeswax/butter will result in a firmer, more paste-like conditioner; more almond oil and/or castor oil will make it softer. Most importantly, remember to always spot test any products—homemade or otherwise—in an inconspicuous area of your leather bag.

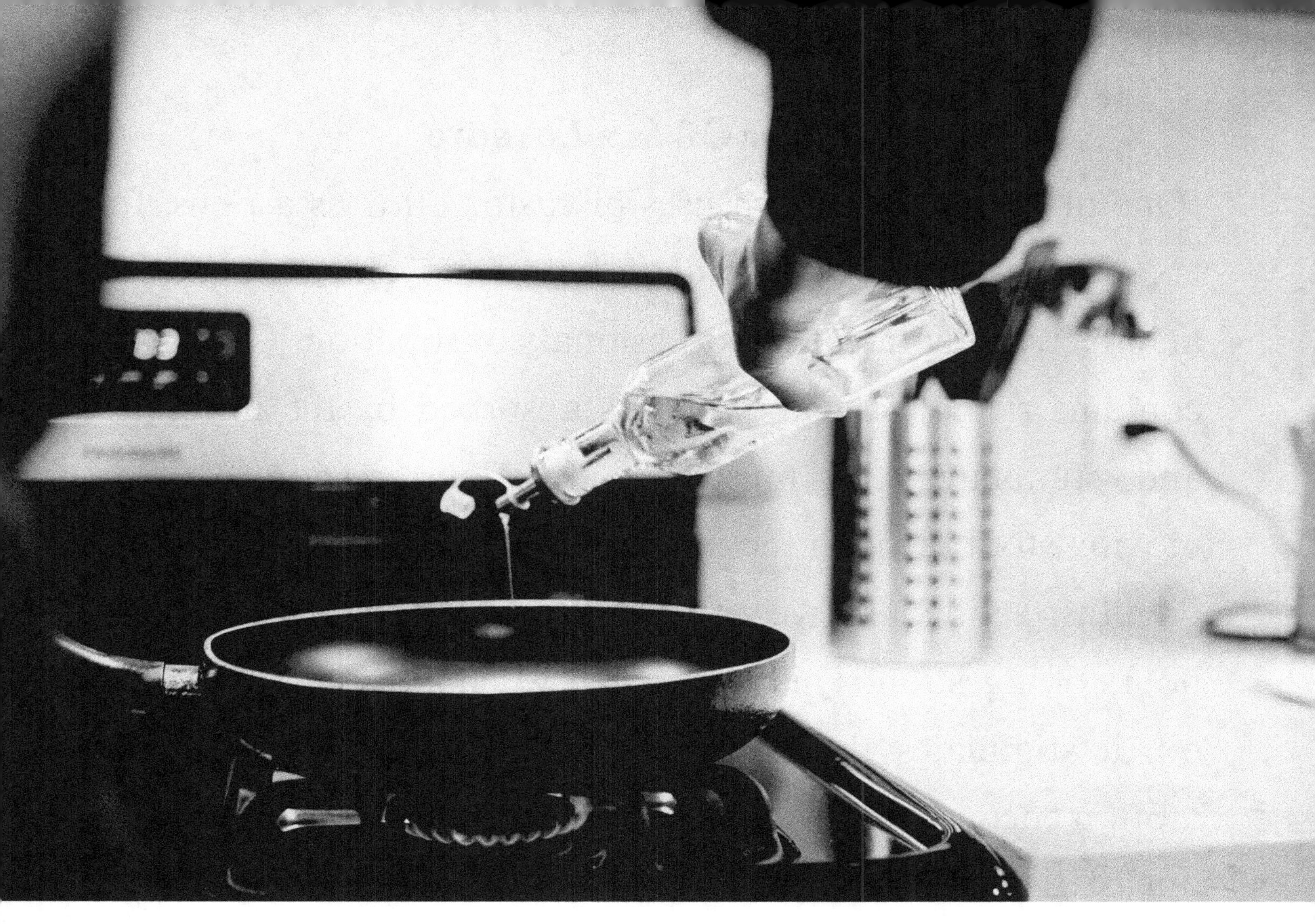

Chapter 10: Castor Oil for Digestive Health: A Natural Laxative and More

Castor oil has been traditionally used as a natural remedy for digestive issues, offering gentle relief from constipation and supporting detoxification processes in the body. In this chapter, we will explore two major ways in which castor oil can enhance digestive health: as a laxative and as a liver detox support through castor oil packs.

Castor Oil as a Laxative

One of the oldest known uses of castor oil is as a powerful laxative. Its ability to stimulate bowel movements makes it an effective treatment for occasional constipation. Castor oil contains ricinoleic acid, which is absorbed by the intestines and stimulates the muscle contractions responsible for moving stool through the intestines. This effect makes castor oil a fast-acting laxative, often producing results within a few hours of ingestion. This means that when a person drinks the oil, it stimulates the bowel to move more. This increased motion encourages the stool to pass through the intestine and out of the rectum. It is advised to use caster oil sparingly because it is a stimulant laxative. Using stimulant laxatives for extended periods may eventually cause the bowel muscles to stop working properly.

Although castor oil can relieve constipation, it can also cause nausea and vomiting as a side effect. Anyone taking castor oil for constipation should be cautious, as it is possible they will become nauseous.

Dosage

People describe the very distinct taste of castor oil as similar to petroleum jelly. The oil is very thick, making it hard to swallow. Some manufacturers add castor oil to other preparations to make it easier to drink. Anyone planning to take castor oil preparations for constipation should always read the label to make sure they are taking the proper dose. A typical dose is around 15 milliliters (ml), which is equal to about half an ounce or 3 teaspoons.

Some people mix castor oil with another liquid or flavored drink to counteract the strong odor and flavor, including:

- fruit juice
- milk
- soft drink
- water

How long does it take castor oil to work?

Castor oil typically causes a bowel movement to occur in 2 to 3 hours. However, it may take up to 6 hours to work for some people. Due to the delayed effects of castor oil, avoid taking it before bedtime.

Cautions

Castor oil is not appropriate for certain groups of people, as it might pose a health risk in specific instances. The Food and Drug Administration (FDA) of the United States categorizes castor oil as a class of drug that, if taken by a pregnant woman, may be harmful to the fetus or result in congenital defects. The hazards of consuming castor oil during pregnancy significantly exceed the benefits.

People with the following symptoms should also avoid castor oil:

- rectal bleeding
- strong, sudden stomach pain
- symptoms of appendicitis
- symptoms of a blocked intestine, such as an inability to pass gas and vomiting
- vomiting

Castor oil should be used as a short-term solution for constipation. Taking castor oil to assist every bowel movement can have serious complications

How to Use:

- **Dosage:** For adults, the recommended dose of castor oil as a laxative is 1-2 tablespoons. Children may take 1-2 teaspoons depending on age and weight, but it is always best to consult a healthcare provider before use.

- **Instructions:** Take the recommended amount of castor oil on an empty stomach, preferably early in the day. Castor oil can have a strong taste, so mixing it with a little juice can help make it more palatable. Expect a bowel movement within 2 to 6 hours after ingestion.

Castor Oil Packs for Liver Detox Support

In addition to its laxative properties, castor oil can be used topically in the form of castor oil packs to support liver detoxification. The liver is a key organ in the body's detox system, and castor oil packs can enhance its function by improving circulation and lymphatic drainage in the area. Do you wake up in the middle of the night and then have a terrible time getting back to sleep? In traditional Chinese medicine, waking between the hours of 1 and 3 AM correlates with the "time of the liver," a cycle in which your liver, the body's largest detox organ, is highly active. By waking, and especially not being able to fall right back to sleep, it may be the liver giving you a sign that it needs a detox of its own.

There's a lot you can do to give your liver some love and help it with detoxifying. Using a castor oil pack placed on the skin over the liver is a time-honored tradition. Many schools of traditional medicine have used castor oil to help support optimized liver function, to improve detoxification and hormonal balance, and to reduce inflammation in the liver.

How to Use a Castor Oil Pack:

Supplies:

- Castor oil
- Large piece of unbleached natural wool or cotton flannel
- Old bed sheet and old towels
- Heating pad or hot water bottle
- Quart-sized glass mason jar
- Tongs

How to:

- Fold your piece of flannel into thirds to make three layers.
- Place the folded flannel in the large mason jar and add a few tablespoons of castor oil, giving the oil time to seep in. Continue to add castor oil a few tablespoons at a time until the cloth is thoroughly soaked.
- Castor oil can stain, so be aware of your surroundings and cover any surfaces (bed, chair, etc.) with old sheets or towels.
- Plug in a heating pad or fill a hot water bottle.

- Carefully remove flannel from jar with tongs and place over liver.
- On top of the flannel, place a towel. Lay a plastic bag over the towel, and place the heating pad on the bag to prevent oil from staining or clinging to the heating pad.
- Relax for 30-60 minutes. You can practice deep breathing, pray, meditate, listen to a podcast, or just close your eyes and let your mind wander.
- After the desired time, remove the pack and return the flannel to the glass container. Store in the fridge.
- Use a natural soap to remove any castor oil left on the skin.
- Drink some water or tea to help you stay hydrated after doing this to support detox.

Benefits of Castor Oil Packs:
- Improved digestion and elimination by stimulating liver function.
- Relief from bloating and abdominal discomfort.
- Enhanced lymphatic circulation and toxin removal.

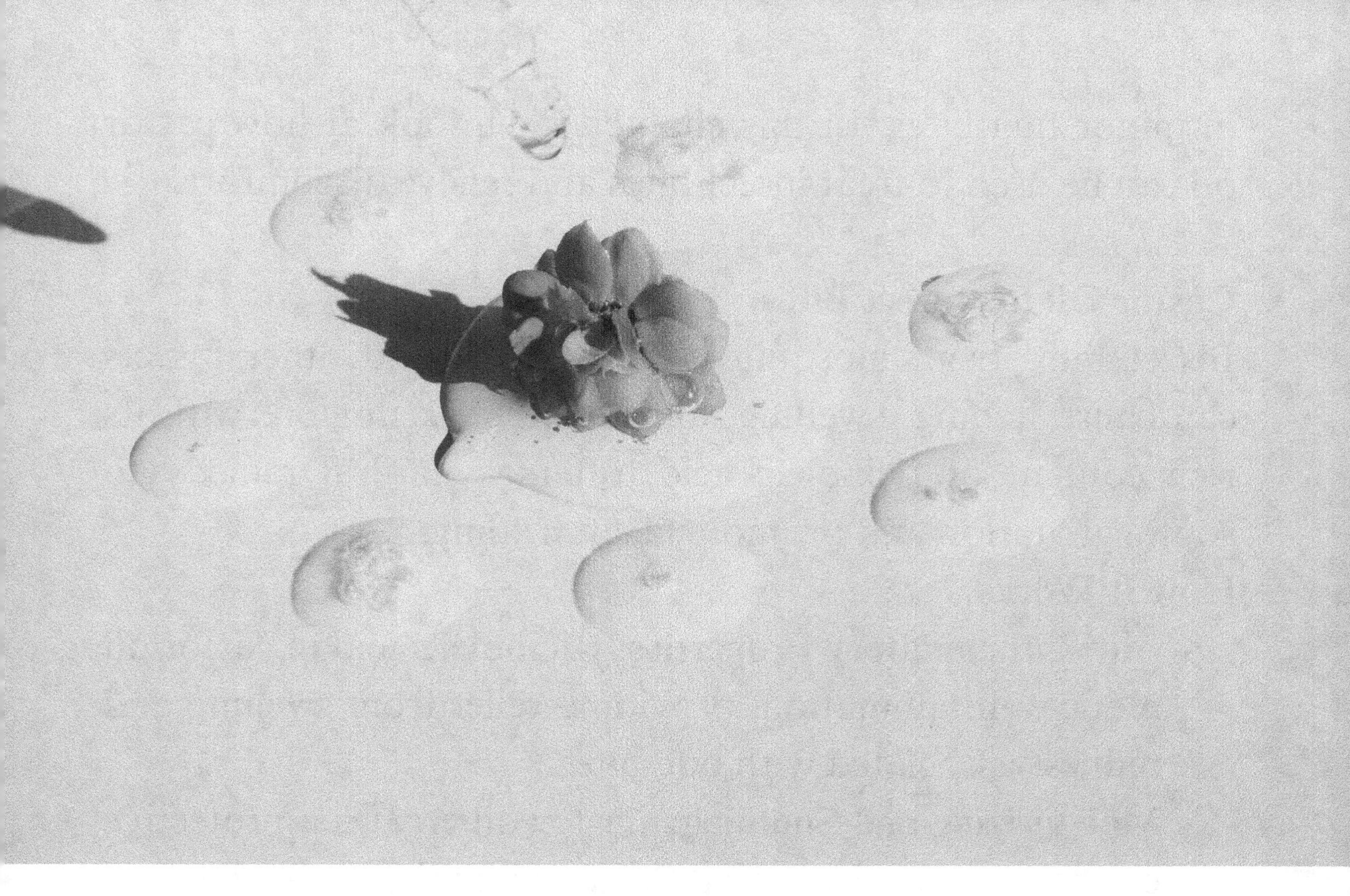

Chapter 11: Castor Oil for Bug Bite Relief and Pest Control: Natural Solutions for Home and Garden

Insect bites can cause irritation, itching, and swelling, but castor oil's soothing and anti-inflammatory properties make it an excellent remedy for quick relief. Castor oil is one of the finest natural insect repellents because it includes the extremely poisonous protein component called ricin. Castor oil has a long history of use as an insect repellent and is a common component in natural bug sprays. It is also known for its antibacterial properties, which help prevent infection in minor bug bites. In this chapter, we'll look at how castor oil can be used to treat insect bites and relieve discomfort.

Castor Oil for Insect Bites

Insect bites from mosquitoes, ants, bees, and other insects can cause itching, swelling, and redness. Castor oil, with its rich content of ricinoleic acid, offers a natural remedy to soothe irritation and promote faster healing.

How It Works:

- **Anti-inflammatory Properties**: Ricinoleic acid in castor oil reduces inflammation, providing relief from swelling and redness associated with bug bites.
- **Moisturizing and Soothing:** Castor oil creates a protective barrier on the skin that locks in moisture and calms itching.
- **Antibacterial:** Castor oil also has mild antibacterial properties that can prevent infection in minor bug bites.

Castor Oil For Mosquito Repellent

According to research, castor oil can significantly diminish mosquito vectors in both their immature and adult stages of development. Plant-based natural oils are widely used for their potent antibacterial, insecticidal, and antifungal properties. Castor oil has the ability to kill insects, including cockroaches and mosquitoes. In pest management and control, castor oil is an effective alternative to pesticides, especially when it comes to controlling cockroaches, termites, and mosquitoes.

Benefits Of Castor Oil For Mosquito Bites

1. Castor oil is one of the finest natural insect repellents because it includes the extremely poisonous protein component called ricin. Castor oil has a long history of use as an insect repellent and is a common component in natural bug sprays.

2. It can be used with essential oils that naturally ward off insects like fleas, ticks, and mosquitoes, such as lavender, lemongrass, and citronella. Although it might not be as powerful as the potent chemicals in aerosol insect spray, using natural bug spray won't be harmful to you or the environment. To sum up, castor oil works well on its own to kill mosquitoes, cockroaches, and other insects.

3. Castor oil keeps mosquitoes at bay. It works extremely well when blended with other mosquito repelling essential oils.

4. Castor oil helps heal mosquito bites. It has strong antibacterial and anti-inflammatory properties to help heal mosquito bites.

Recipe Of Castor Oil Mosquito Repellent

Castor oil works as an all-natural and non-toxic insect repellent. When combined with other potent insect repelling essential oils, the benefits are doubled. Here is how you can make your own DIY mosquito repellent:

Supplies:

- Water: 1.5 Tablespoon
- Castor Oil, 1 Teaspoon
- Thyme Essential Oil, 10 Drops
- Geranium Essential Oil, 5 Drops
- Lemongrass Essential Oil, 10 Drops

How to:

- Take a spray bottle and add water and castor oil to it.
- Now, add all the essential oils one by one.
- Cover the bottle with the cap and give it a good mix by shaking it thoroughly.
- Spray the mixture on your body or at any place as and when required.

Caster Oil for Pest control

Wild animals can pose a problem in the home garden. Mole hills pop up overnight, skunks dig up prized plants in search of grubs, and squirrels unearth your bulbs and render them useless for the bloom season. One way to minimize the damage that naturally occurs when animals forage is to use castor oil as pest control. How does castor oil repel animal pests? It seems the bitter taste and the unpleasant smell are the keys. Just as children had to hold their noses to take the stuff back in the day, so too, our animal friends are sickened by the ripe odor and bitter taste.

The Benefits of Castor Oil in Pest Control

Environmentally Friendly: Castor oil is a natural, renewable resource, making it an eco-conscious choice for pest control. Its use in pest management products minimizes the impact on the environment and helps promote a healthy ecosystem.

Non-Toxic: Castor oil is safe for use by people, pets, and other wildlife, in contrast to many chemical-based pest control methods. This makes it the perfect option for gardeners and homeowners who care about the environment, their families, and their pets.

Effective Against a Various of Pests: Research has shown that castor oil works well as a repellent and deterrent against a range of pests, such as gophers, moles, voles, and other rodents. Moreover, it can aid in the prevention of insects, including spider mites, aphids, and whiteflies.

Biodegradable: Castor oil is a natural substance that breaks down easily in the environment, leaving no harmful residues behind. This makes it a more sustainable option compared to synthetic chemicals that can persist in the environment and negatively impact soil, water, and wildlife.

Multi-Functional: Castor oil has the ability to improve soil health and supply plants with vital nutrients, in addition to its ability to fight pests in your garden. Its organic lubricating qualities can even aid in keeping garden tools from rusting.

Simple Application: Whether in the form of sprays, granules, or pellets, castor oil-containing pest control treatments are usually simple to apply. This makes keeping unwanted pests out of their plants and landscapes a simple task, even for inexperienced gardeners.

Castor Oil in the Garden as a Pesticide

Castor oil won't kill animal pests, but it will repel them. To harness the effect, you need to apply castor oil directly to the soil. The formula will work for a week or so, even in the rainy season. Weekly applications are the most effective at controlling animal damage in the garden. These animals get diarrhea from consuming castor oil, so they do everything to get away from the oil. They are sure to stay away from the garden and start searching for a new place to thrive.

Recipe Of Castor Oil Mosquito Repellent

Supplies:

- 2 tablespoons of dishwashing liquid
- ¼ cup of caster oil
- 4L of water

How to:

- Mix two tablespoons of any dishwashing liquid with a quarter cup of castor oil.
- Dilute the two tablespoons of the castor oil and dishwashing liquid mixture in a gallon of water.
- Spray it all over the infested areas.

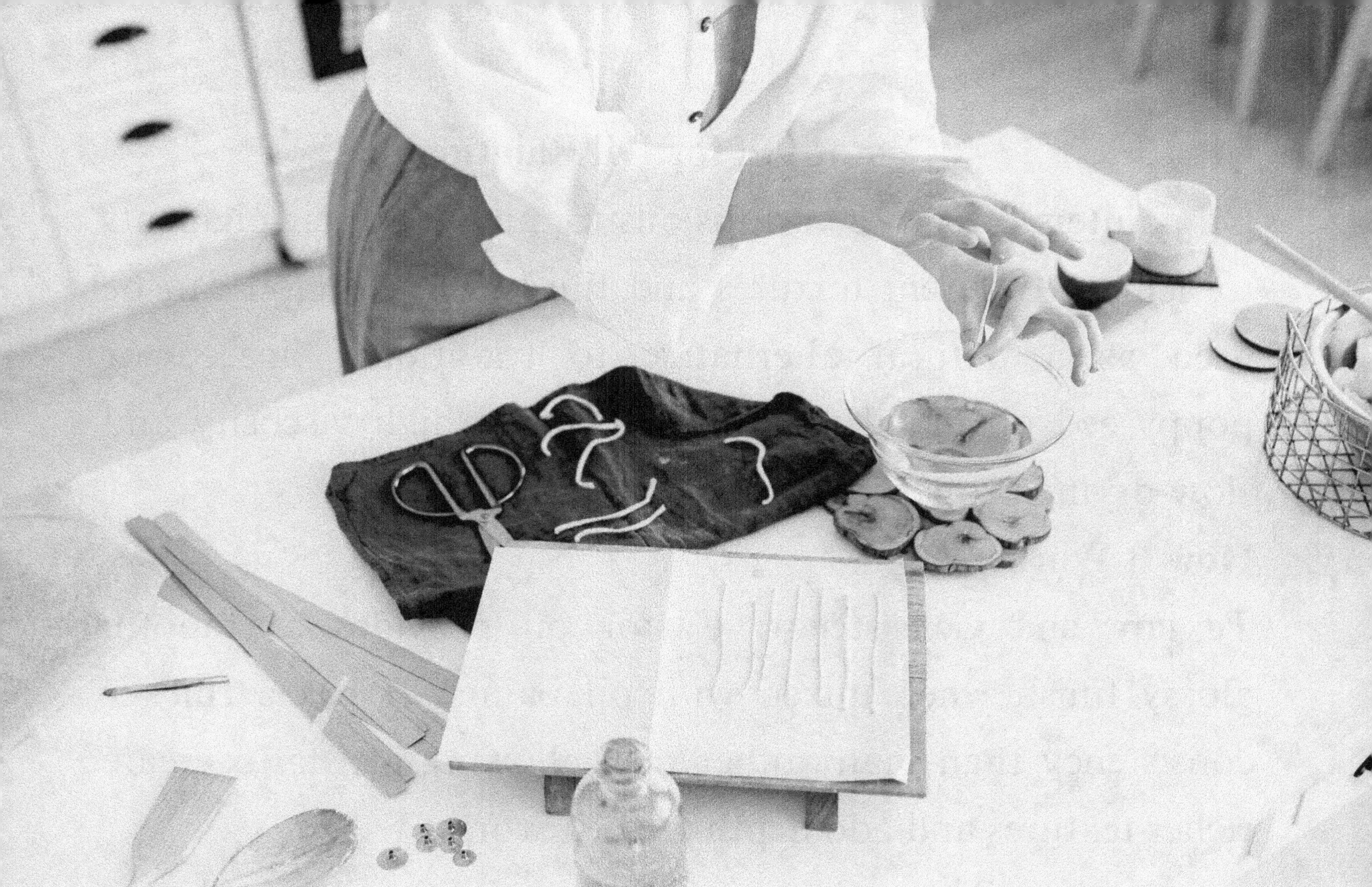

Chapter 12: Creative Uses of Castor Oil: Enhancing Art and Craft

Beyond its uses in health and wellness, castor oil has surprising applications in the world of art and craft. Its unique texture and viscosity make it a valuable medium in oil painting, where it can serve as a natural additive. A lot of the paint business depends on raw materials that can make the finished product better in terms of quality and performance. Castor oil is very important in this situation. This chapter will explore how castor oil can be used in oil painting to enhance the texture and longevity of artwork.

Castor Oil for Oil Painting

Oil painters often use various oils to mix with their pigments to achieve different textures and finishes. Castor oil can be used as a natural alternative to traditional linseed or poppyseed oil in oil painting due to its high viscosity and slow-drying properties.

How It Works:

Texture and Consistency: Castor oil provides a smooth, glossy finish when mixed with oil paints. It has a thicker consistency than many other oils, allowing artists to create richer textures and add depth to their work.

Slow Drying Time: Castor oil's slow drying time makes it ideal for blending and layering colors over an extended period. This gives artists more flexibility when working on detailed sections of their paintings.

Durability: Castor oil helps to protect and preserve paintings by forming a durable film on the surface. This ensures the longevity of the artwork while maintaining the vibrancy of the colors.

Improving Paint Flexibility: Paint for walls needs to be able to stretch and shrink with changes in temperature without cracking. Because castor oil makes the paint flexible, it can handle these changes without losing its shape. This quality is very important for keeping painting walls looking nice, especially in places where the temperature changes a lot.

- Mix castor oil with oil paints in small amounts to modify the texture and drying time. Artists can experiment with the ratio of oil to paint to achieve their desired effect.
- Use a brush to apply the castor oil-mixed paint onto the canvas, blending it as needed. Allow for extra drying time, as castor oil takes longer to set than traditional oils.

Additional Tip:

For artists who prefer a glossy finish, castor oil can be applied as a final varnish to oil paintings. A thin coat can enhance the sheen and protect the artwork from dust and grime.

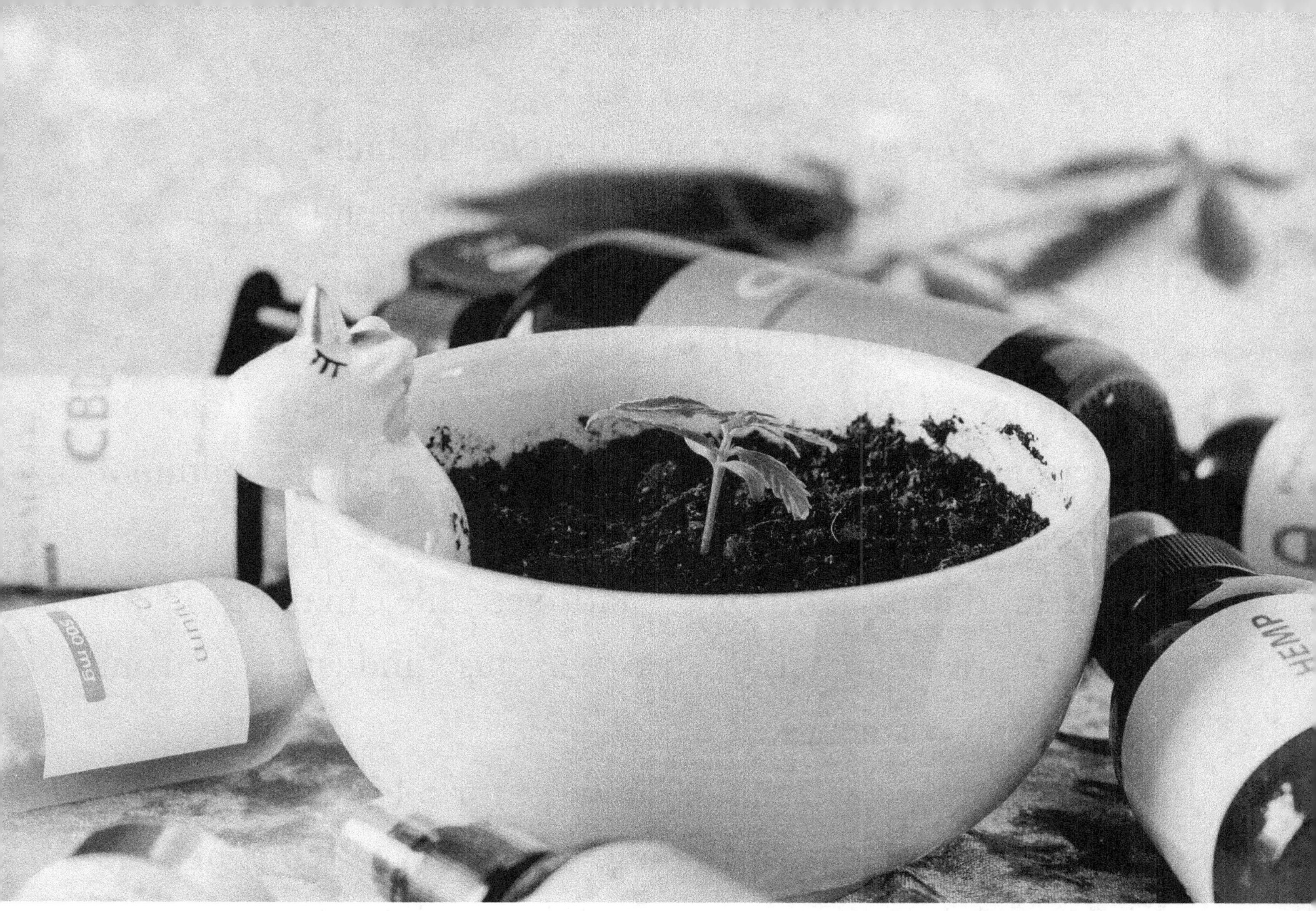

Chapter 13: Castor Oil in Eco-Friendly Products: Paving the Way for Sustainable Health and Beauty

As the world moves toward sustainability and eco-friendly solutions, castor oil has emerged as a versatile ingredient in various environmentally conscious products. Its renewable nature and wide range of applications make it an ideal component in sustainable manufacturing. In this chapter, we will explore how castor oil is being used to create sustainable products and its potential role in shaping the future of health and beauty.

Castor Oil for Sustainable Products

As the world seeks alternatives to petroleum-based and environmentally harmful products, castor oil has emerged as a renewable and sustainable resource with a wide range of applications. Unlike many other crops used for oil production, castor plants are hardy and require minimal resources, making them an eco-friendly choice. The oil itself is biodegradable, non-toxic, and versatile, making it an attractive raw material for various industries, from bioplastics to cosmetics.

In this section, we will explore how castor oil is used to create sustainable products, including its role in reducing the environmental impact of plastics, industrial materials, and consumer goods.

1. Castor Oil in Bioplastics

Bioplastics are a sustainable alternative to traditional petroleum-based plastics, which contribute significantly to pollution and environmental degradation. Castor oil is a valuable feedstock for producing certain types of bioplastics, particularly polyamides and polyurethanes, which are used in everything from automotive parts to electronics and packaging materials.

How Castor Oil Helps Produce Bioplastics

- **Biodegradability:** Castor oil-derived bioplastics are often biodegradable, meaning they break down more easily in the environment compared to conventional plastics. This reduces the accumulation of plastic waste in landfills and oceans.

- **Renewability:** Castor oil is sourced from plants that can be grown year after year, making it a renewable resource, unlike petroleum, which is finite.

- **Lower Carbon Footprint:** The production process for castor oil bioplastics generates fewer greenhouse gas emissions compared to the production of traditional plastics.

Applications of Castor Oil Bioplastics:

- **Automotive Industry:** Castor oil-based polyamides are used in making lightweight automotive components, such as fuel lines and engine covers, which reduce vehicle weight and improve fuel efficiency.

- **Packaging:** Castor oil can be used in the production of eco-friendly packaging materials. These materials provide an alternative to single-use plastics, offering a biodegradable solution for consumer products.

- Textiles and Footwear: Several eco-conscious brands use castor oil-based materials in textiles for clothing and footwear. These materials are not only sustainable but also durable and lightweight.

Example:

Castor oil-based polyamides are used in high-performance materials for the automotive, electronics, and consumer goods industries. Companies like Evonik and Arkema are industry leaders in this regard. These businesses are looking into novel ways to incorporate castor oil into various applications that have historically relied on goods derived from petroleum.

2. Green Lubricants and Industrial Applications

Beyond bioplastics, castor oil is also used in the production of eco-friendly lubricants and industrial products. Conventional lubricants are often made from petroleum, and their widespread use in machinery, vehicles, and household appliances contributes to pollution. Castor oil's unique chemical structure, which includes a high percentage of ricinoleic acid, makes it an ideal candidate for developing biodegradable, non-toxic lubricants.

Advantages of Castor Oil Lubricants:

Biodegradable: Unlike synthetic lubricants that persist in the environment and can be toxic to wildlife, castor oil-based lubricants break down naturally and pose no harm to ecosystems.

High Viscosity: Castor oil is highly viscous, meaning it remains effective at high temperatures and pressures, making it suitable for heavy-duty machinery, automotive engines, and industrial equipment.

Non-Toxic and Safe: Because castor oil is naturally derived and non-toxic, it is a safer option for use in household products, personal care items, and industrial applications that may come into contact with humans or animals.

Applications of Castor Oil-Based Lubricants:

- **Machinery and Engines:** Castor oil lubricants are used in industrial machines, vehicles, and even in aviation engines due to their stability under extreme conditions.

- **Household Products:** In household items like hair clippers, razors, and bicycles, castor oil lubricants are a natural, safe alternative to synthetic oils.

- **Personal Care Products:** Many eco-friendly personal care products, such as hair oils, are made using castor oil because of its lubricating properties and skin-friendly nature.

Example:

Castrol and other lubricant manufacturers have developed castor oil-based formulations for high-performance engine oils, especially for motorsports, where biodegradable options are gaining popularity due to increasing environmental regulations.

3. Castor Oil in Sustainable Cosmetics and Personal Care

The health and beauty industry is undergoing a revolution toward sustainability, and castor oil is becoming a key ingredient in eco-conscious beauty products. Its nourishing properties make it ideal for skin and hair care, while its renewability and non-toxicity appeal to brands and consumers looking to minimize environmental impact.

Why Castor Oil is Perfect for Sustainable Beauty:

- Natural and Effective: Castor oil is rich in fatty acids and vitamin E, making it an effective moisturizer and hair conditioner. It is used in everything from natural soaps to organic makeup removers.

- No Harmful Chemicals: Many traditional beauty products contain synthetic chemicals and preservatives, which can harm the environment. Castor oil offers a natural alternative, free from harmful additives.
- Fair Trade and Organic Sourcing: Castor oil is often sourced from small-scale farms that use organic methods, ensuring that its production does not contribute to soil degradation or pollution. Many companies are also focusing on fair trade castor oil, ensuring that the farmers receive fair compensation.

Examples of Castor Oil Beauty Products:
- Skincare: Castor oil is a common ingredient in moisturizers, lip balms, and cleansing oils due to its ability to hydrate and protect the skin.
- Hair Care: Castor oil is known for its ability to promote hair growth and is often used in leave-in conditioners, hair serums, and scalp treatments.
- Makeup: In eco-friendly makeup, castor oil serves as a base for products like mascara, eyeliner, and lip gloss, providing a natural shine and smooth application.

Example:
Castor oil is now a staple in many brands' product lines, like Weleda and Kreyol Essence, which offers consumers organic, ethically sourced, and efficacious beauty products that support their environmental objectives.

4. Castor Oil in Eco-Friendly Packaging and Zero-Waste Initiatives

As consumers and companies alike aim to reduce waste, castor oil is being used in innovative ways to create sustainable packaging and support zero-waste initiatives. Plastic packaging is a major contributor to environmental pollution, but castor oil-based alternatives offer a biodegradable and renewable option.

How Castor Oil Helps Reduce Packaging Waste:

Biodegradable Plastics: Castor oil-derived plastics can be used to create packaging that biodegrades more quickly than conventional plastics, reducing the accumulation of waste.

Eco-Friendly Coatings: Castor oil is used in producing eco-friendly coatings for paper and cardboard packaging, providing water-resistant properties without the need for harmful chemicals.

Zero-Waste Beauty Packaging: Many beauty and personal care brands are turning to castor oil as a component in their packaging to create zero-waste products, where even the packaging can be composted or easily recycled.

Examples:

Castor oil is used to create biodegradable packaging for cosmetics, food products, and even medical supplies.

Lush and other zero-waste beauty brands are utilizing castor oil in their packaging materials, ensuring that their products are as sustainable as their contents.

Castor Oil in the Future of Health and Beauty

As consumers become more aware of the environmental and health impacts of the products they use, there is a growing shift toward natural, sustainable, and ethically sourced ingredients in the health and beauty industry. Castor oil, with its long history of use in traditional medicine and natural beauty remedies, is emerging as a key ingredient in the future of sustainable beauty and personal care. In this section, we will explore how castor oil is influencing current trends in health and beauty, its potential to shape the industry's future, and why it is increasingly favored by both consumers and brands.

1. The Rise of Clean Beauty and Castor Oil's Role

"Clean beauty" is a growing movement that prioritizes products free from harmful chemicals, synthetic additives, and environmental toxins. Consumers are seeking beauty solutions that are effective yet safe for both the body and the environment. Castor oil is a natural fit for this movement due to its gentle, non-toxic nature and versatility in formulation.

Why Castor Oil is a Clean Beauty Staple:

- Natural Origin: Castor oil is 100% plant-based, derived from the seeds of the castor plant. This makes it an ideal choice for consumers looking for non-synthetic, organic ingredients in their beauty routines.
- Free from Harsh Chemicals: Unlike many traditional beauty products that use preservatives, parabens, sulfates, and artificial fragrances, castor oil is naturally pure and does not require chemical additives to be effective. Its ability to stay stable for long periods reduces the need for preservatives.
- Hypoallergenic: Castor oil is suitable for sensitive skin types and is less likely to cause allergic reactions compared to synthetic ingredients commonly found in mainstream beauty products. Its gentle nature makes it a popular ingredient in formulations designed for delicate skin, such as baby products and sensitive skincare lines.

How Clean Beauty Brands Use Castor Oil:

- **Moisturizers and Serums:** Castor oil's emollient properties make it a key ingredient in hydrating lotions and facial serums. It locks in moisture, leaving the skin soft and smooth without clogging pores, making it ideal for both dry and oily skin types.
- **Hair Care Products:** Castor oil is used in hair oils, conditioners, and leave-in treatments to promote healthy hair growth and repair damaged strands. Its fatty acids nourish the scalp and strengthen hair follicles.
- **Natural Makeup:** Castor oil is often included in the formulation of natural makeup products like lip balms, mascara, and foundation. It provides a smooth texture, enhances product longevity, and adds a natural shine to cosmetics without the need for synthetic oils or waxes.

Trend Prediction:

More businesses will use castor oil as a foundational base in their formulations as well as an active ingredient as the clean beauty trend continues to expand. The popularity of multipurpose, minimalist cosmetic products is a great fit for castor oil's adaptability, which lets businesses use fewer ingredients while still producing high-quality goods.

2. Sustainable Sourcing and Fair Trade Castor Oil

The beauty business is starting to prioritize sustainability; thus, ethical ingredient sourcing is becoming more and more important. Because castor plant cultivation has little environmental impact, especially in arid and semi-arid locations, castor oil stands out as a sustainable resource. Additionally, the promotion of fair trade guarantees that the production of castor oil supports nearby farmers and their communities.

Sustainability of Castor Oil Production:

- **Low Environmental Impact:** Castor plants thrive in dry, degraded soils that are not suitable for other crops. This reduces the need for irrigation and synthetic fertilizers, making castor oil production more eco-friendly compared to other oil crops like palm or soybean.
- **No Deforestation:** Castor oil is not associated with the large-scale deforestation issues that plague other oil-producing industries, such as palm oil. This makes it a more ethical choice for brands looking to avoid ingredients linked to environmental destruction.

Fair Trade Initiatives:

Economic Empowerment: Many castor oil-producing regions are in developing countries, and fair trade programs ensure that small-scale farmers receive fair compensation for their labor. This helps improve local economies and promotes ethical business practices in the global supply chain.

Transparent Sourcing: Consumers are increasingly demanding transparency in how ingredients are sourced. Brands using fair trade castor oil can offer their customers peace of mind, knowing that their beauty products contribute to positive social and environmental impacts.

Example:

Companies such as The Body Shop and Kreyol Essence are leading the way in obtaining fair trade and organic castor oil. These businesses promote the benefits of castor oil for skin and hair as well as for the communities that grow it, emphasizing its ethical and sustainable production.

3. Castor Oil's Role in Multi-Use and Zero-Waste Products

In line with the growing demand for minimalist and zero-waste beauty products, castor oil's versatility allows it to play a central role in formulating products that serve multiple functions, reducing the need for excessive packaging and waste. As consumers look for ways to simplify their beauty routines while reducing their environmental footprint, castor oil-based products are leading the way in this trend.

Multi-use Beauty Products:
- One Ingredient, Multiple Benefits: Castor oil can serve as a moisturizer, makeup remover, lip balm, and hair conditioner, all in one. Its ability to perform various functions makes it a key ingredient in multi-use products, which are increasingly popular with consumers who want to declutter their beauty cabinets.
- Minimalist Skincare: In the age of minimalist beauty, consumers are looking for products that offer maximum efficacy with minimal ingredients. Castor oil's hydrating and healing properties allow it to be used as the main ingredient in simple yet effective skincare regimens.

Zero-Waste Packaging:
- Sustainable Packaging Solutions: Many brands are turning to zero-waste initiatives, reducing or eliminating plastic packaging in favor of eco-friendly alternatives. Castor oil-based products can be packaged in biodegradable containers or offered in refillable formats to align with zero-waste goals.
- Solid Beauty Bars and Balms: Castor oil can be used in solid skincare and haircare bars, reducing the need for plastic bottles. These solid formats, such as cleansing bars or hair

conditioning balms, are ideal for travel and are packaged in paper or tin, further reducing environmental impact.

Trend Prediction:

The future of beauty will likely see an increase in products that serve multiple functions and are packaged sustainably. Castor oil's adaptability makes it a natural choice for these types of products, as it aligns perfectly with the minimalist, eco-conscious values that are driving the industry forward.

4. Castor Oil's Role in Innovative Future Beauty Technologies

As science and innovation continue to advance, castor oil's unique chemical composition is being studied for use in cutting-edge beauty and personal care technologies. Whether through its application in nanotechnology for enhanced delivery systems or its potential use in regenerative skincare, castor oil's versatility makes it an attractive ingredient for future beauty innovations.

Nanotechnology and Enhanced Delivery Systems:

- **Castor Oil in Skincare Formulations:** Scientists are exploring the use of castor oil in nanotechnology-based delivery systems, which can enhance the absorption of active ingredients into the skin. Castor oil's small molecular size allows it to penetrate the skin barrier effectively, making it an ideal carrier oil for delivering nutrients deep into the skin.

- **Liposome Formation:** Castor oil's structure is being explored for the development of liposomes—tiny spherical vesicles used in advanced skincare to encapsulate and deliver active ingredients like vitamins and peptides into the skin more efficiently.

Regenerative Skincare:

- Cellular Repair and Anti-Aging: Castor oil's fatty acids and antioxidant properties make it a promising candidate for anti-aging and regenerative skincare products. As the demand for non-invasive, natural anti-aging solutions grows, castor oil is being studied for its potential to repair damaged skin cells and stimulate collagen production, helping to reduce the appearance of fine lines and wrinkles.

Example:

Castor oil is being used in formulas by brands like Drunk Elephant and The Ordinary because of its bioactive and skin-compatible qualities. These businesses are taking advantage of castor oil's capacity to deliver additional active ingredients deep into the skin as well as its benefits for deep hydration.

Weekly Breakdown of the Detox Plan

In this section, we will explore a comprehensive 30-day detox plan that leverages the unique properties of castor oil to cleanse and rejuvenate different systems in the body. This detox is designed to be gentle and holistic, supporting the liver, digestive system, skin, lymphatic system, joints, and muscles. Each week is focused on a different aspect of health, with practical applications of castor oil through topical treatments, internal use, and recipes for detox support. This plan aims to help individuals achieve a full-body reset by the end of the four weeks.

Week 1: Gentle Liver and Digestive Cleanse

The first week of the detox focuses on supporting the liver and digestive system. Castor oil has long been known for its ability to aid digestion and detoxify the liver, one of the body's primary organs for filtering toxins.

How to Use Castor Oil Packs for Liver Detox:

- **Materials Needed:** Wool or flannel cloth, castor oil, plastic wrap or a towel, and a heating pad.

- **Instructions:** Soak a piece of cloth in warm castor oil and apply it directly over the liver area (right side of the abdomen, just below the rib cage). Cover the cloth with plastic wrap or a towel to avoid staining, and place a heating pad over it. Leave it on for 45-60 minutes. Use this pack 3-4 times during the week to stimulate liver detoxification and improve circulation.

Recipe: Castor Oil Lemon Detox Tonic (For Occasional Internal Use)

While castor oil can be taken internally for digestive cleansing, it should be used sparingly to avoid overuse.

Supplies:

- 1 tablespoon of cold-pressed castor oil
- Juice of 1 fresh lemon
- 1 cup of warm water

How to:

- Mix the castor oil with lemon juice and warm water.
- Drink this mixture on an empty stomach once or twice during the week to help promote gentle bowel movements and liver detoxification.

This tonic helps to clear the digestive tract while supporting the liver's natural cleansing processes.

Week 2: Skin and Lymphatic System Detox

During week two, the focus shifts to detoxifying the skin and lymphatic system. The lymphatic system plays a crucial role in eliminating toxins and waste from the body. Dry brushing combined with castor oil massages can enhance lymphatic drainage, and castor oil's ability to penetrate deeply into the skin makes it an excellent carrier oil for detoxification.

Dry Brushing and Castor Oil Massage for Lymphatic Drainage:

- **Dry Brushing:** Use a dry brush with natural bristles to brush your skin in circular motions before showering, starting from the feet and moving upwards toward the heart. This helps to stimulate the lymphatic system and exfoliate dead skin cells.
- Castor Oil Massage: After dry brushing and showering, apply castor oil to the skin using gentle, circular motions. Focus on areas like the neck, armpits, and groin where lymph nodes are concentrated. This massage helps support lymph flow and detoxification.

Recipe: Detoxifying Castor Oil Body Scrub

This body scrub helps to exfoliate the skin, boost circulation, and detoxify the body through the skin's pores.

- 1/2 cup of cold-pressed castor oil
- 1/2 cup of sea salt or Epsom salt
- 5-10 drops of essential oils (optional: lavender, tea tree, or eucalyptus for detox support)

How to:

- Mix the castor oil with the salt and essential oils.
- In the shower, gently massage the mixture onto your skin in circular motions, focusing on areas prone to buildup like the arms, legs, and back.
- Rinse off with warm water.

Use this scrub 2-3 times during the week for exfoliation and detoxification.

Week 3: Joint and Muscle Detox

In week three, the detox plan focuses on relieving tension, soreness, and stiffness in the joints and muscles. Castor oil's anti-inflammatory properties can help alleviate discomfort and aid in the removal of toxins from these tissues. Castor oil packs can be used for deeper detoxification of the joints and muscles, especially for those who suffer from chronic pain or inflammation.

Applying Castor Oil Packs to Sore Muscles and Joints:

- **Instructions:** Similar to the liver pack, apply a cloth soaked in warm castor oil directly onto sore muscles or joints. Cover with plastic wrap or a towel, and place a heating pad on top. Leave it on for 45-60 minutes to allow the castor oil to penetrate deeply and reduce inflammation.

Recipe: Castor Oil and Ginger Anti-Inflammatory Pack

Ginger enhances castor oil's anti-inflammatory properties, making this pack especially useful for sore or inflamed areas.

- 2 tablespoons of cold-pressed castor oil
- 1 teaspoon of freshly grated ginger or ginger powder
- Wool or flannel cloth, plastic wrap, and a heating pad

How to:

- Mix the castor oil and ginger together.
- Soak the cloth in the mixture and apply it to the sore area.
- Cover with plastic wrap and apply heat with a heating pad for 45 minutes to an hour.

This pack can be applied to joints, muscles, or even the lower back for relief from pain and stiffness.

Week 4: Full-Body Rejuvenation

The final week of the detox is about rejuvenating the entire body. After detoxifying the liver, skin, lymphatic system, and muscles, this week focuses on incorporating castor oil into both internal and external routines to promote overall vitality.

Incorporating Castor Oil in Diet and Skincare for Overall Vitality:

- **Diet:** Optionally, small amounts of castor oil can be incorporated into your diet to promote digestive health. It's important to use this sparingly, as castor oil can have a strong laxative effect if overused. Consider using it once or twice during the week in small doses, such as 1 teaspoon mixed into smoothies or warm beverages.

- **Skincare:** Continue with castor oil massages and scrubs to support skin health and rejuvenation. Castor oil's rich fatty acids nourish the skin, helping to improve elasticity, reduce the appearance of scars, and promote a healthy glow.

Recipe: Castor Oil and Peppermint Oil Bath for Relaxation and Detox

This bath helps soothe tired muscles, promote relaxation,

This bath helps soothe tired muscles, promote relaxation, and aid in detoxification through the skin.

Supplies:

- 2 tablespoons of cold-pressed castor oil
- 5-10 drops of peppermint essential oil
- 1 cup of Epsom salts

How to:

- Mix the castor oil with the essential oil and Epsom salts.
- Add the mixture to a warm bath and soak for 20-30 minutes.
- Focus on deep breathing and relaxation while the castor oil and Epsom salts help draw out toxins and soothe your muscles.

Conclusion: Reviving Castor Oil for Modern Wellness

As we come to the end of this journey through the world of castor oil, it's clear that this ancient remedy is more than just an elixir from the past. Castor oil's rich history, diverse applications, and scientific backing demonstrate its value as a powerful tool for promoting health and well-being in our modern lives. Let's recap some of the key takeaways from this book and why castor oil deserves a place in your everyday health routine.

Key Takeaways:

- **A Rich History of Healing:** Castor oil has been used for thousands of years, from ancient Egypt to Ayurvedic medicine, for its healing and nourishing properties. This longstanding history speaks to its effectiveness in promoting health across many cultures.

- **Versatility Across Health and Beauty:** From skincare to digestive health, castor oil offers a wide range of benefits. It can soothe inflammation, promote detoxification, enhance beauty routines, and even alleviate common ailments like joint pain, menstrual cramps, and skin irritations.

- **Scientific and Anecdotal Evidence:** Modern research supports the age-old wisdom surrounding castor oil. Scientific studies highlight its antimicrobial, anti-inflammatory, and laxative properties, while generations of anecdotal evidence showcase its effectiveness in natural remedies.

- **Sustainable and Eco-Friendly:** In a world increasingly conscious of sustainability, castor oil stands out as an eco-friendly choice. Its low environmental impact, ethical sourcing opportunities, and biodegradability make it a perfect fit for today's demand for natural, sustainable products.

- **Customizable and Accessible:** Whether you are making your own skincare products, relieving pain with a castor oil pack, or using it in a hair treatment, castor oil is easy to incorporate into your daily life. Its affordability and accessibility mean that almost anyone can benefit from this versatile oil.

Incorporating Castor Oil into Everyday Health:
With its multitude of uses, castor oil can become a staple in your daily routine. Whether you're looking to enhance your skin and hair care, support your digestive system, or address specific health concerns like joint pain or skin conditions, there are numerous simple ways to integrate castor oil into your life.

- **Skincare Routine:** Use castor oil as a moisturizer, makeup remover, or ingredient in homemade scrubs to maintain glowing, healthy skin.
- **Digestive Support:** On occasion, castor oil can be used as a natural laxative to ease constipation or support detoxification.
- **Pain Relief:** Castor oil packs can be applied to sore muscles and joints to reduce inflammation and promote healing.
- **Hair and Scalp Care:** Regularly massaging castor oil into the scalp can encourage hair growth, combat dandruff, and nourish dry, brittle hair.

Encouragement for the Future
In a world filled with synthetic products and quick-fix solutions, castor oil offers a return to natural, sustainable, and time-tested remedies. By incorporating this versatile oil

into your everyday routine, you're not only embracing a holistic approach to wellness, but you're also tapping into the wisdom of generations who have used castor oil to nurture their bodies.

As you move forward, consider making castor oil a regular part of your self-care and wellness rituals. Its benefits are broad and long-lasting, and with each use, you are reconnecting with the power of nature's remedies. Whether for beauty, health, or household uses, castor oil can be your partner in achieving a healthier, more balanced life.

Revive the power of castor oil, and let this elixir play a central role in your journey to wellness.

REVIEW

Dear Reader,

Thank you so much for reading "The Castor Oil Elixir." I hope it has provided you with valuable insights and practical tips to improve your health and well-being.

If you enjoyed the book or found it helpful, I would greatly appreciate it if you could leave a review on Amazon. Your feedback will not only help others discover the benefits of castor oil but will also support me in reaching more readers like you.

To leave a review, simply visit the book's page on Amazon and share your thoughts. Your review means the world to me and will help others in making informed decisions!

Thank you for your support!

Warm regards,

Jenna Jones

Author and Health Advocate